NAB RESIDENTIAL CARE/ ASSISTED LIVING EXAM STUDY GUIDE—2ND EDITION

Client/Resident Services Management
Dorothy M. Witmer, EdD, RN

Human Resources Management
Robert Van Dyk

Leadership and Governance
Diane K. Duin, PhD

Physical Environment Management
Lisa J. Schaaf Yehl, MHSA, LNHA, and Delvin Zook

Financial Management
Christian A. Mason

Prepared by
National Association of Long Term Care Administrator Boards, Inc. (NAB)

Edited by
Mary Helen McSweeney-Feld, PhD

Production Manager
Mark Wright

Web-based Enhancement
Fusion Productions

Printed in 2010
Copyright © 2007 (revised 2010) by National Association of
Long Term Care Administrator Boards, Inc.

ISBN 0-9635064-7-1

All inquiries should be addressed to:
National Association of Long Term Care Administrator Boards, Inc.
1444 I Street, NW
Suite 700
Washington, DC 20005
www.nabweb.org

Acknowledgement

The second edition was updated in 2010. NAB wishes to acknowledge the work of
Heather Anderson, who updated the current edition.

CONTENTS

FOREWORD

Members of the National Association of of Long Term Care Administrator Boards (NAB) have worked diligently since 1997 to create, support, and update the only national competency exam for residential care/assisted living managers. This study guide has likewise been updated to assist you in preparing for the new examination.

As part of the framework for describing the development and use of the residential care/assisted living examination, it is important first to describe NAB's role. NAB is the national not-for-profit association serving state-level entities that license, credential, and regulate administrators of organizations across the long term care continuum. Our goal is to enhance the effectiveness of our members to protect the public interest. We accomplish our goal by working with our 50 state affiliates and the District of Columbia, regarding examination, licensure, and regulatory issues. The primary functions of NAB are the development and implementation of the residential care/assisted living administrator examination; the development and implementation of the nursing home administrators examination; approval of long term care baccalaureate/advanced degree programs; reviewing and preauthorizing continuing education programs for states and organizations; and continuing support related to changing federal requirements.

Residential care/assisted living (RC/AL) has grown rapidly over the past two decades because its emphasis is on innovation in living arrangements and service delivery. In addition, as a consumer-driven service option, residential care/assisted living is an attractive alternative for many seniors exploring safe,

nonmedical housing and care. Because this profession is growing so rapidly, it is important to assure the public that adequately trained and knowledgeable individuals manage these types of communities. It is obvious that resistance to additional regulations in RC/AL is strong. However, it has become widely accepted that there is now a need for an examination to address minimum competency issues. The development and implementation of this examination are through the effort of many states and NAB, and are meant to provide a proactive approach to the concerns of licensing boards where applicable, as well as consumer groups and industry leaders.

NAB and Professional Examination Service (PES), the organization that oversees development and implementation of the examination, have taken careful steps to ensure that this examination was originally designed and continues to be designed completely free of any linkage to the nursing home administrators examination. This effort has lead to ever-increasing support of this national examination.

Because each state takes a different approach to long term care administrators, especially in the RC/AL profession, I'd like to provide a brief background about the creation of the national RC/AL examination and this study guide. In the early 1990s, several states requested that NAB assist them with the development of an examination to gauge minimum competency in the areas of residential care/assisted living management. During a three-year period, the exam development process took place. An initial task force assembled participants from state and federal regulatory agencies, national service organizations, and industry. In addition, the American

College of Health Care Administrators, the Assisted Living Federation of America, the American Health Care Association, the American Association of Homes and Services for the Aging, and the National Association of Residential Facilities (which later merged with the Assisted Living Federation of America) all provided important input in the formative steps. The task force agreed on a definition of the professions, conducted a job analysis survey using 2,300 practicing RC/AL administrators, and defined the domains of practice for administrators in this field.

After the task force completed the preceding preliminary steps, it started the exam development process actually in 1997. Many practicing administrators and scholars from around the country participated in writing questions that were then used to create the first RC/AL examination. Following development of this examination, a standard setting workshop was held to set the score for passing. The score setting process is paramount to developing a successful and relevant examination. The job analysis was updated in 2005.

Since 1997, several additional states have begun using the RC/AL examination to establish minimum competency for candidates entering the RC/AL profession. NAB's RC/AL Examination Committee meets on an ongoing basis to develop new items, review and revise exams, and act as a sounding board for issues or ideas that may surface. We believe it is essential that administrators practicing in the RC/AL field participate in the development of this examination. Should you or someone you know be interested in participating in this ongoing examination development process, please contact NAB for consideration. Although we realize that an entry-level examination does not provide all the answers, it does play an important role in helping ensure that entry-level RC/AL administrators have basic essential knowledge and information.

We hope that examination candidates find this study guide valuable as they prepare for taking the examination. We encourage you also to review other resource materials referenced in this study guide. We have taken great steps to limit our reference list to a manageable number to assist the candidate in reasonably preparing to take and pass this examination successfully. Residential care/assisted living is a rapidly changing environment as part of the long term care continuum, and it is essential that candidates have a good knowledge base and understanding of the needs and desires of those we serve. The developing social, medical, financial, and human aspects of RC/AL necessitate that candidates know the field far beyond the limited scope of this study guide.

On behalf of NAB, I would like to acknowledge the tremendous contribution of each author and the many individuals who assisted with reviews. It is only through the efforts of our volunteers that we are able to produce this quality study guide. Editor Mary Helen McSweeney-Feld worked innumerable hours to pull the guide together with the help and support of NAB President & CEO Randy Lindner and Production Manager Mark Wright. We are proud to offer this second edition of the study guide to meet the needs of our member states, consumers, advocates, and professionals seeking to ensure quality care and services for our constituents.

My deep thanks to all,

Margaret McConnell
NAB Chairman

INTRODUCTION

What the Study Guide Offers

NAB publishes this second edition of its study guide to help you prepare for its Residential Care/Assisted Living Administrators Examination. The study guide offers you a valuable package of information that covers the knowledge, tasks, and skills reflected in the exam.

This second edition recognizes revisions in NAB's domains of practice for RC/AL administrators that were approved by the NAB Board of Governors in 2005. These domains identify current consensus about the knowledge and skills required to be an effective administrator in these facilities and guide the preparation of questions for this examination. The revised domains of practice also reflect the growth of the residential care/assisted living (RC/AL) industry and important management concepts, philosophies, and legislation that affect the delivery of services to residents.

To make the study guide as effective as possible, NAB has enhanced this book with an online learning tool. The concepts presented in the Web enhancement are based on the book, but the computer-based format gives you an opportunity to learn in an interactive manner. NAB decided to produce the study guide in this combined format to help you use all your senses in the learning process. The online version replaces the CD-ROM that accompanied the first edition.

What the Study Guide *Isn't*

Please keep in mind that this examination study guide is *not* a textbook. The material presented here is not a collection of everything you could ever know as a residential care/assisted living administrator. Reviewing this material will not guarantee that you will pass the examination; however, you will find it extremely useful toward that end.

Rather, the study guide is designed to help you review key concepts and areas of practice. The study guide, like the exam, is aimed at the individual entering the field. It covers topics that represent a baseline of knowledge about the role of an entry-level administrator in an RC/AL environment.

State Requirements Vary

Requirements for RC/AL administrators vary tremendously from one state to the next. Your state might have very basic requirements, or it might have a rigorous set of regulations.

Because each state differs in its approach to RC/AL administrator standards, this study guide can address the administrator's role only from a general perspective. Your education about the knowledge, skills, and tasks of an RC/AL administrator should include serious study of a number of publications. NAB includes a bibliography of such publications in its *RC/AL Information for Candidates Handbook*. The bibliography is updated periodically, so visit the NAB Web site (www.nab-web.org) for a current copy of the handbook.

Additional Resources

The NAB study guide also serves as a gateway to other information. Other organizations and publications are adding to the body of knowledge available to RC/AL administrators who seek to develop their understanding of and abilities in the field. We include references to a number of these other sources.

A Quick Tour of the Study Guide

Chapter 1

The first chapter profiles the National Association of Long Term Care Administrator Boards (NAB) and explains how NAB assists state licensing boards in carrying out their responsibilities.

Chapter 2

Chapter 2 deals with the nature of the RC/AL administrator examination, its structure and content, and how to prepare for the exam and offers some general tips on taking this computer-based test. Candidates should pay particular attention to the test specifications presented here. The test is based on five major subject areas—the domains of practice—that incorporate specific knowledge and skills for an RC/AL administrator.

Chapters 3–8

Chapters 3 through 7 cover the specifics of those domains of practice. One chapter is devoted to each domain: client/resident services management, human resource management, leadership and governance, physical environment management, and financial management. Chapter 8 is on Person-Centered Care in Assisted Living. Each chapter includes a series of practice questions, any references used by the author in writing the chapter, and a glossary of terms.

Using the Practice Questions

None of the practice questions at the end of chapters 3 through 8 will appear on the actual exam. The practice questions simply offer you some experience in answering questions similar to those on the real exam. The practice questions also provide an additional learning opportunity because they are followed with the correct answers and an explanation of each correct answer. By reviewing the rationale for the correct answer, you can verify and reinforce your knowledge of the subject.

Acknowledgments

NAB wishes to acknowledge and thank all the people who helped make this study guide possible. The authors—Diane K. Duin, PhD; Christian A. Mason; Robert Van Dyk; Dorothy M. Witmer; Lisa J. Schaaf Yehl, MHSA, LNHA; and Delvin Zook—worked hard to make this second edition of the study guide a great tool aimed at helping you meet the challenge of the RC/AL administrator exam. They also hope you find this work to be a foundation for your continuing professional growth.

A special word of thanks to those who helped review all or parts of the study guide prior to its printing. Their comments and suggestions were invaluable in refining the finished product. Reviewers included:

Philip S. Brown, MA, LNHA, Executive Director of Asbury Group Homes, Inc., North Carolina

Steven E. Chies, Senior Vice President, Long Term Care Operations, Benedictine Health System, Cambridge, Minnesota

John H. Hogan, Executive Director, Mary's Woods, Lake Oswego, Oregon; Instructor, Health Care Administration Program, Oregon State University

Susan J. Hunter, Executive Director, United Methodist Retirement Center, Salem, Oregon

Joan Johnson, Senior Area Programming Manager, Sunrise Senior Living, Phoenix, Arizona

Keith Knapp, PhD, CNHA, Chief Operating Officer, Christian Care Communities, Louisville, Kentucky

Margaret McConnell, Owner/Administrator, The Charleston, Las Vegas, Nevada, NAB Chairman

Mark P. McConnell, MBA, Owner/Administrator, The Fountains Senior Care, Inc., Reno, Nevada

Sister Phyllis McCracken, SSJ, MS, RN, NHA, President/CEO, Saint Mary's Home of Erie, Erie, Pennsylvania

Louis Rubino, PhD, FACHE, Associate Professor, California State University, Northridge, California

Katherine E.W. Will, PhD, Administrator, Morrison Health Care, Inc., Lancaster, Ohio

Special thanks to Mary Helen McSweeney-Feld, PhD, for her work in editing the book.

NAB appreciates the assistance of Bruce Anderson from Professional Examination Service (PES).

Finally, thank you! Your commitment to learning and improving as a residential care/assisted living administrator means everyone—from your facility stakeholders, to your fellow professionals, and most important, your residents and their families—is enriched and better served. NAB wishes you success and fulfillment in your journey.

CHAPTER 1

ABOUT NAB

The National Association of Long Term Care Administrator Boards (NAB) is a voluntary, nonprofit membership organization comprised of state boards or agencies responsible for licensing long term care administrators. NAB assists these state boards and agencies in carrying out their responsibilities in the original licensure and relicensure of long term care administrators. In pursuit of its mission, NAB engages in activities and programs in four major areas.

The first major area of work is in exam development and administration. Two of NAB's important programs include the development of the national nursing home administrator examination, which the state boards administer to applicants as part of their requirements for a nursing home administrator license, and more recently the development of the national residential care/assisted living (RC/AL) administrator exam, available to states as part of their requirement for RC/AL licensure or as a voluntary competency exam. NAB contracts with a prestigious testing organization, Professional Examination Service, to provide expert guidance and assistance to NAB and its examination committees, to handle the distribution of the examinations, and to score the results.

NAB's second area of focus is in continuing education and standard setting for licensure. NAB recommends to state boards and agencies standards for consideration and adoption. Based on a passing point study, NAB recommends to states the passing score for the licensure examination. NAB also passes curricular guidelines for college and university baccalaureate degree programs in long term care administration. It provides guidelines for

administrator-in-training programs and has established criteria for continuing education programs. As part of its work in continuing education, NAB operates a continuing education review service. When education programs submitted for review meet the NAB criteria, the programs are approved for a specified number of credits.

NAB's third area of emphasis is research. NAB publishes annual reports that contain summary statistics on first-time test takers and on candidates retaking tests. The annual reports also contain demographic data on first-time test takers, such as age, sex, academic preparation, and long term care–related work experience.

To ensure that the NHA and RC/AL examinations keep pace with changes in long term care administration, NAB conducts job analysis studies every five years. The studies determine entry-level practice for long term care administration. One outcome of the studies is the development of revised test specifications for the examinations.

The final major NAB area of focus is publications, including job analyses for nursing home administrators and RC/AL administrators, annual reports, study guides, exam information handbooks, and more. Visit www.nabweb.org for the latest list of NAB publications.

Most of NAB's work is done through its committees, including the Executive, Bylaws, Policies and Procedures, NHA and RC/AL Examination, Education, Continuing Education, Standards of Practice, Marketing and Public Relations, and Budget and Finance committees. Eligible committee participants include the members of state licensing boards and agencies and their executive directors and

1

former members of state licensing boards and agencies who choose to retain their affiliation with NAB by becoming associate members. Subscribing members are also eligible for service on all committees except the examination committees. Faculty members in long term care programs and representatives of other organizations related to the long term care field are eligible for such subscribing membership.

NAB was incorporated in New York on January 13, 1971. The Board of Governors, consisting of one voting delegate from each member jurisdiction, has supervision, direction, and control of the affairs of the organization. The Executive Committee has authority in policies, procedures, and rules established by the Board of Governors to act for the NAB and has charge of its routine affairs in between Board of Governors meetings.

Mission

The National Association of Long Term Care Administrator Boards (NAB) will be the nationally leading authority on licensing, credentialing, and regulating administrators of organizations along the continuum of long term care.

Code of Ethics

The following principles of professional conduct are developed for members of boards that license long term care administrators. The code of ethics is established to provide guidance in relationships with licensees and potential licensees, other health professionals, regulatory agencies, and the public.

As a Board member that licenses Long Term Care Administrators, I pledge:

1. To strive for the constant improvement of care and services for residents in health care facilities with emphasis on the preservation of the honor and dignity of each individual.
2. To work toward the elevation of the profession of long term care administration through quality educational offerings, research and statistical studies, publications and professionals, regulatory agencies, and the public.
3. To treat all licensees and applicants on an impartial basis and respect the rights, privileges, and beliefs of others regardless of race, creed, color, sex, age, handicap, or any other discriminatory factors.
4. To recognize my position, as a member of this board, as a position of public trust and to keep confidential all information learned regarding licensees and applicants and that my conduct will be guided by all applicable regulations and professional standards.
5. To agree not to receive or agree to receive, directly or indirectly, any payment, gift, or gratuity for any activity related to the duties or responsibilities of the board unless so provided by law.
6. To constantly seek to improve my professional knowledge and skills of the profession of long term care administration.
7. To work to improve the effectiveness of the licensure system and the board's accountability to the public.

CHAPTER 2

ABOUT THE EXAMINATION

The overall objective of this study guide is to help those individuals seeking to enter the practice of <u>residential care/assisted living</u> <u>(RC/AL) fa</u>cility administration to prepare for the NAB RC/AL administrators examination. The best way to prepare for the examination is to gather as much information as possible so that you have an idea of what to expect before the actual test administration.

The information in this study guide should not be used alone or as a substitute for textbooks or other reference sources that contain the knowledge an administrator requires to function on the job. This study guide is intended as a supplemental aid in preparing for the examination.

Examination Development

The NAB licensing/entry-level competency examination helps to protect the public by ensuring that entry-level residential care/ assisted living administrators and executive directors have mastered a specific body of knowledge and can demonstrate the skills and abilities essential to competent practice within the profession.

State boards or agencies that currently license RC/AL administrators and executive directors establish the requirements for licensure. (Refer to NAB's Web site at www.nab-web.org to determine which states require or offer the RC/AL licensure examination.) In states that require licensure, any individual who wishes to enter or continue in the practice of RC/AL administration must meet the standards established by his or her state or jurisdiction to qualify for or maintain an occupational license.

The examination is developed by a committee appointed by NAB, with the assistance of Professional Examination Service (PES), a not-for-profit testing organization whose major focus is the development, validation, and administration of examinations in health and health-related fields. The NAB RC/AL Examination Committee, composed of experts in the field of RC/AL administration, meets on a regular basis to review and update the examination.

The examination is based on a role delineation and validation study, also referred to as a job analysis. To conduct the job analysis, a panel of RC/AL facility administration experts convened to outline the major areas of practice, work-related tasks, and the knowledge and skills that an administrator must have to perform his or her job. To ensure that the outline developed by the panel actually described the work of an entry-level RC/AL administrator, the outline was sent to a sample of RC/AL administrators across the country for validation. The panel requested that the validation sample review the outline for accuracy and rate the major areas of practice and the task statements in terms of importance, frequency of performance, and criticality. The ratings of the validation sample were used to develop the content and test specifications (blueprint) for the examination.

Item Development

Items (questions) for the examination are written by RC/AL facility administrators throughout the United States. Each item undergoes a <u>rigorous re</u>view process that includes screening and editing by content experts to ensure subject matter accuracy and relevance, and editing by PES for clarity and conformity to psychometric principles. The items are then independently reviewed by the NAB RC/AL Examination Committee before they are used in the examination.

Practice Questions

Each of the five domain-specific chapters in this study guide includes a brief practice test. Be sure to work through the sample test questions after you have read a chapter. Doing so will enhance your understanding and retention of the material.

Information for Candidates

To guide exam candidates through the application process, and to provide more in-depth information about the exam and the computer-based testing process, NAB publishes a free *RC/AL Information for Candidates* handbook. With the assistance of PES, the handbook is periodically updated.

The *RC/AL Information for Candidates* handbook covers these topics:

- Frequently asked questions
- Test specifications
- Testing procedures
- State exam
- About NAB's national computer-based test
  - Completing an application form
  - When the application is completed
  - Scheduling the examination(s)
- The computer-based test experience
- Rescheduling, extensions, withdrawals, and no shows
- Sample test questions
- Examination bibliography
- Diagnostic score report of results form
- Interstate reporting service form
- Candidate request for special accommodations form
- Publications available from NAB

Reading the handbook is a vital step for all examination candidates. In addition to providing guidance and insights, it provides the forms a candidate needs at different points during the process. Copies can be downloaded for free from the Exams section of NAB's Web site (www.nabweb.org).

DOROTHY M. WITMER, EdD, RN, has practiced as a professional nurse for more than 40 years, including Air Force nursing, acute care, long term care, community health, and nursing and allied health education. She has a bachelor's degree in nursing from Villanova University, a master's degree in community health from the University of Illinois, and a doctoral degree in education from the University of Idaho. In recent years, Dorothy has concentrated on care of the elderly in long term care settings and has developed programs in Idaho for educating nursing home and assisted living healthcare care professionals. Dorothy has her own consulting business, Healthcare Education and Training. She received the Life Enrichment Award from the Idaho Health Care Association in 2006 and the Nursing Legend Award in 2004 for her many contributions to nursing and healthcare.

CHAPTER 3

CLIENT/RESIDENT SERVICES MANAGEMENT

Dorothy M. Witmer, EdD, RN

Introduction

In the United States, the number of residential care/assisted living (RC/AL) facilities is increasing at a rapid rate. RC/AL represents one part of the long term continuum of care for older adults that lies somewhere between independent living centers and nursing homes. As more people live longer, the need for RC/AL facilities is expected to escalate. Influencing the increase is the change in demographics: aging people who need assistance with care are no longer able to turn to their family members as they have been able to do in years past. Many family members who would be available to care for loved ones now work or have moved away. Elderly people still want to be as independent as possible and want to age in a comfortable environment more like home (Allen 2004). RC/AL facilities offer this kind of housing option.

According to the National Center for Assisted Living (NCAL), the philosophy of assisted living "emphasizes the right of the individual to choose the setting for care and services. Assisted living customers share the risks and responsibilities for their daily activities and well-being with a staff geared to helping them. . . ." (NCAL Customer Information) The philosophy also contains a belief that these facilities allow residents to age in place; residents can stay at the facility until the care staff can no longer provide for their health, safety, and well-being. The RC/AL administrator is responsible for integrating the philosophy into services provided and ensuring that the personnel who deliver the services abide by it.

A key concept in resident services provision in RC/AL facilities is **person-centered care.** Person-centered care optimized quality of life and quality of care with the goal of enhancing resident function and well-being. Relationships among staff, residents and families are at the heart of person-centered care. It is transformation from a paternalistic/materialistic model of care to a consumer-directed model that honors elders' life experiences, interests, routines of daily living through relationships. An understanding of person-centered care is imperative for today's RC/AL administrators as this approach is becoming more and more recognized as the gold standard. Refer to Chapter 8 Person-Centered Care for more information. An example of this is when the resident wants to sleep late and bathe later in the day, but the staff are told all baths must be given in the morning starting at 6:00 A.M. Person-centered care requires changes in how a facility operates and in the behaviors of staff. These changes produce a change in the culture of the facility that is hard to accomplish but that adds a great deal to the quality of life of residents.

RC/AL administrators typically describe their facilities as being run according to the **hospitality model** of resident care and services. Hospitality has many definitions depending on who you ask. Merriam-Webster defines *hospitality* as being hospitable, which means "friendly, kind, and solicitous." Another meaning is "favoring the health, growth, and comfort, etc., of new arrivals," a meaning that immediately relates to the RC/AL industry. Hospitality also includes good customer service—those behaviors that personnel in an organization or business undertake during their interactions with customers—in all aspects of resident care.

Evidence of hospitality begins before a resident moves into the facility. Marketing the facility includes outlining the special services and features a person can expect to access as a resident and assuring potential residents that the staff is kind, friendly, and caring (Waye 2005). When the standards of hospitality are applied, the results should be high-quality care and services that satisfy residents.

The administrator who communicates with residents frequently and routinely walks around the facility to talk with staff members can learn how well hospitality standards are being applied. Obviously, RC/AL staff must adopt hospitality standards and apply them daily. Periodic audits of service areas help the administrator keep track of how services are rendered and how hospitality is implemented.

Ways to evaluate how the hospitality standards are working include distributing surveys to residents and family members and forming a resident committee that reviews complaints. One aspect of hospitality is predicated on providing a fast response to complaints and reports of services that need to be fixed. Daily communication with residents and staff continues to be very important because communicating directly and immediately with residents who are dissatisfied and concerned staff can help to reduce the number of complaints. Residents want to know something is being done to correct a situation, and staff need to know how they can help. Hospitality is key to the longevity of the RC/AL facility.

The Aging Process and Profile of RC/AL Residents

Residents who choose to live in RC/AL facilities require assistance with activities of daily living. They have one or more chronic illnesses that have reduced their capacity to function without assistance. There is growing recognition that chronic illness is a major healthcare problem in the United States. Its prevalence and the costs associated with it are expected to rise with the increasing number of elderly people. Most of the residents in RC/AL facilities are elderly. This section concentrates on the changes that aging people experience with a focus on the physiological, psychosocial, and mental changes, as well as related diseases and conditions. Administrators should have some understanding of the aging process and its related changes to anticipate the kinds of services residents will require.

Physiological Changes of Aging

Physiological changes that aging people experience can be described by reviewing the many systems of the body. Body systems work together so that one system may affect another. Each person ages differently. Some people seem very old at 80 years, whereas others are quite active and live independently at that age. This section also describes diseases and conditions that are known to occur in younger populations that reside in RC/AL facilities. Administrators should have a basic knowledge of physiologic changes and diseases of aging so that they can plan, implement, and evaluate prevention and care measures.

In general, as people age, all body organs tend to decrease in size and the systems of which they are a part decrease in function. Changes that occur in nine body systems and some of the consequences that result from these changes, including common related diseases, can be found in Table 3.1. Neurological disorders are discussed here because of the incidence of cognitive impairment and dementia in so many older people.

Neurological-related disorders and disease. Parkinson's disease is a neurological disease characterized by slowness and weakness of voluntary movement, rigidity, and tremors,

Table 3.1 Physiological Changes of Aging		
Body System	**Changes**	**Consequences**
Integumentary—Skin	Decreased cells, moisture, elasticity, body hair, subcutaneous fat, blood flow, and perspiration; increased rigidity of connective tissue	Skin becomes dry; tears and bruises easily; less tolerance for heat and cold; susceptible to infection; dermatitis
Circulatory	Decreased cardiac output, enzyme action on heart, heart rate, and ability of heart to return to normal after illness; increased tendency for high blood pressure; blood vessels accumulate fatty deposits; decrease in blood return to the heart	Insufficient blood supply to vital organs during illness; blood pressure drops with changes in posture; mental confusion; poor circulation to extremities; swelling of feet and legs; cold hands and feet; arteriosclerosis, coronary heart disease
Respiratory	Lungs become restricted by rib cage; rib cage size increases; lung tissue becomes more rigid; decrease in respiratory strength; lungs do not expand fully; lower lung expands less, upper lung more	Dyspnea on exertion; less oxygen and carbon dioxide exchanged; breathing more shallow; less effective cough reflex; tendency for lung diseases; emphysema, pneumonia
Musculoskeletal	Decreased muscle fibers and tissue, muscle strength; increased waste products in muscle (lactic acid, carbon dioxide); muscle cells accumulate fat and collagen; bones become porous and lose bone mass; calcium leaves the bone; tendency for spinal curvature; decreased elasticity and ability to move joints	Inactivity produces loss of strength in limbs; postural changes; unstable gait; more falls; stiffness; osteoporosis; fractures occur more often; arthritis, osteoarthritis
Digestive	Teeth loosen and gums recess; loss of taste buds; decrease in enzyme actions, hydrochloric acid (HCL), peristalsis, ability to tolerate fat, gag reflex, and sphincter controls	Tooth loss; false dentures; poor appetite; nutritional deficiencies; increase in gum disease and food intolerances; choking more frequently; constipation increases; less protein intake; tendency for hiatus hernia; gastroesophageal reflux disease (GERD)
Endocrine	Decrease in cells, size of glands, gland secretions, ability to adapt to stress because of decreased adrenaline, decreased thyroid secretions	Tendencies for hypothyroidism, diabetes, autoimmune diseases, and lowered resistance to diseases; body temperature decreases; females prone to vaginal infections; males prone to slower ejaculations

continued

9

Table 3.1 Physiological Changes of Aging *(continued)*		
Body System	**Changes**	**Consequences**
Urinary	Decrease in size of kidneys, functional cells, vascular circulation to kidneys, urine produced and eliminated, filtering function of kidneys; decreased tone of urinary muscles and ability to control flow of urine	Less ability of kidneys to eliminate medications; tendency for acid–base imbalance of body fluids and electrolytes; tendency for nocturia, frequency of urination, urinary infections, urinary retention, and incontinence; less time between sensation to void and need to void
Reproductive	Females: decrease in size of ovaries, uterus, and amount of hormonal secretions; lining of vagina becomes thinner Males: prostate enlarges; decrease in size of testes; ejaculations slowed; sexual function and activity continues; more time required for satisfaction	Females: tendency for pruritis (itching) and irritation of vagina; tendency for prolapse of uterus after many pregnancies; cancer Males: problems with urination as a result of obstruction from enlarged prostate; cancer
Neurological	Decrease in brain weight, neural cells, psychomotor reaction time, blood flow to the brain, and in all sensory perceptions: hearing, vision, touch, taste, sense of balance; memory loss; plaques form in brain tissue	More time needed for activities of daily living (ADLs) and learning; slower reactions to stimuli; tendency for falls; adjustments and devices needed for senses; cognitive impairment; strokes

especially of the arms. It is a degenerative disease that may be completely debilitating in older people. Afflicted individuals are subject to falls.

Organic/chronic brain syndrome is a term applied to conditions that include dementia and that are characterized by progressive, irreversible degeneration. People with these brain syndromes have impaired cognition, memory loss, and personality changes and cannot think abstractly.

Dementia in the Elderly

The Alzheimer's Association through a consensus process with 26 other organizations developed dementia care practice recommendations for assisted living residences.

The following information is excerpted from these practice recommendations[1].

Each person with dementia is a unique individual possessing distinct interests, capabilities, and needs. They are able to experience meaning in their daily lives, opportunities to do new things, and enjoyment among other capacities. As their dementia progresses, individuals with dementia will experience changes in their abilities, interests and needs making regular assessments essential. For individuals with dementia residing in assisted living, their quality of life depends largely on the quality of the relationships they have with their direct care staff.

---

[1] Reed, P.R., Tilly, J. (2005). Dementia Care Practice Recommendations for Assisted Living Residences and Nursing Homes. Alzheimer's Association, Chicago, IL.

Good dementia care in assisted living includes: regular assessment of a resident's abilities; interdisciplinary service planning including strategies for addressing behavioral, physical and communication changes; appropriate staffing patterns; and a nurturing and engaging environment that fosters community. Optimal care occurs within a social environment that supports the development and maintenance of healthy relationships between staff, family and residents. Staff find out how best to serve each resident by learning as much as possible about them including their life story, preferences, interests and needs. Staff use this information to develop 'person-centered' strategies designed to help optimize each resident's capabilities and function.

Staff need initial and ongoing training, support, and supervision that empowers them to develop skills to care for individuals with dementia. Staff need to be able to identify potential triggers for a resident's behavioral and emotional symptoms by using environmental and behavioral strategies to prevent or modify the impact. Staffing patterns should ensure that residents with dementia have sufficient assistance to meet their needs and participate in the daily life of the residence. Consistent staffing assignments helps to promote relationships between staff and residents.

The physical environment is especially important for individuals with dementia as dementia challenges their ability to understand new environments. A positive physical environment has recognizable areas for daily life such as sleeping, bathing, toileting, clothes storage, and dining among others. The optimal environment feels comfortable and familiar as their home would providing opportunities for privacy, pleasant sounds such as music, and minimizes negative stimuli such as loud noises and overhead paging. The physical environment also needs to be safe and secure and provide access to the outdoors while maintaining security over elopement. Residents with a history of elopement will need special focus and planning to manage this behavior safely.

Individuals with dementia may need assistance ensuring that they maintain sufficient consumption of appropriate foods and fluids. The disease can impact on their perceptions of hunger and thirst. Towards the later stage of dementia individuals may experience difficulty with swallowing, an inability to feed themselves due to impairments in functional mobility, altered perceptions of smell and taste, and an inability to recognize items such as dining utensils. Good dementia care provides for mealtimes that are pleasant and enjoyable to maximize a positive dining experience. Effective staff approaches to ensuring a positive dining experience include opportunities for residents to be involved such as setting the tables, stimulating olfactory senses with the smells of food, removing mealtime distractions, serving foods and drinks that the residents like, and being sensitive to the need for compatible dining companions.

Some individuals with dementia are very active, such as those that walk constantly, requiring special attention to ensuring their diets contain sufficient calories. Foods higher in nutrient density, calories and protein should be included in their daily diets. Only in extreme circumstances should liquid supplements be considered. Residents need opportunities to drink fluids throughout the day. Fluids can be incorporated into activities such as serving cups of water routinely after programs.

Meaningful activities are the foundation of good dementia care because they help residents maintain their functional abilities and provide opportunities for involvement in the community that are important for belonging and feeling part of the community. Good dementia care entails the need for planned activities as well as spontaneous ones. For example, every encounter or exchange between residents and staff is an opportunity for socializing and a chance to engage with a resident. Meaningful activities include a number of domains: physical movement; mental stimulation; social interaction; spiritual participation and/or fulfillment; recreational

11

interests such as watching a baseball game, and cultural and traditional celebrations such as birthdays and holidays. Group size and lengths of time for engagement need to be tailored to each individual.

The engagement of residents is not the sole responsibility of the activity staff. Every staff member has the responsibility and should ensure opportunities to interact with residents daily.

Managing pain for individuals with dementia can be challenging and under-recognized since their communication skills are compromised. One of the challenges is assessing and communicating with them about their pain experience and about the side effects of medications. Treat pain as a 'fifth vital sign' by routinely assessing and treating it in a formal, systematic way similarly as one would treat blood pressure, pulse, respiration and temperature.

Prevention of pain is the first defense against it. Some pain can be addressed through the regular use of medications. Offering medications 'as needed' though may not be sufficient treatment for many residents. Observing residents when they move may uncover pain issues that may not occur when they are at rest. There are many pain scales and tools available and staff may want to experiment with various types to determine which ones work most effectively for residents. All staff should be involved in pain management by being trained to record their observations and report signs of pain in residents to their supervisors.

Many individuals with dementia move about in ways that may appear aimless but which are often purposeful. This movement is known as wandering. Wandering may be a behavioral expression of a basic human need such as for social contact, or a response to physical discomforts, environmental irritants, or psychological distress. Wandering can be helpful when it provides stimulation, mobility, or social contact. Physical movement helps strength preservation, prevention of skin breakdown and constipation, and enhancement of mood.

Wandering is problematic when the movement includes exit seeking behavior from the safety of the assisted living home without an appropriate companion. This eloping behavior may be following old habits, such as thinking they are leaving for work, or they may be drawn outside by a sunny day. Exit seeking without an appropriate companion is dangerous and can result in injury and potentially death.

People who wander persistently are the source of 80 percent of elopements. About 45 percent of these incidents occur within the first 48 hours of admission to a new residence. The unfamiliarity of the new environment may make individuals with dementia more confused. Staff need to be especially focused during the first week helping a new resident feel comfortable and at home, and be alert for exit seeking behavior.

Administrators have the responsibility to ensure that the assisted living community's policies and procedures support the above referenced aspects for quality dementia care. Two well-known resources for additional information about good dementia care include the Best Friends model (bestfriendsapproach.com) and Dawn Brooker, "Person Centered Dementia Care: Making Services Better."

Profile of RC/AL Residents

RC/AL services are typically determined by the needs and preferences of residents. However, not all services are provided by RC/AL facilities to all residents. For example, some facilities require that persons are ambulatory or need little assistance with ambulation, and are not incontinent. Some facilities provide services for specific populations, such as those who are mentally ill, those who are mentally retarded/developmentally disabled (MR/DD), residents with dementia/Alzheimer's disease, substance abusers, or the frail elderly.

A survey recently conducted by the American Association of Homes and Services for the Aging (AAHSA), American Speech-Language-Hearing Association (ASHA), Assisted Living Federation of America (ALFA), National Center for Assisted Living (NCAL), and the National Investment Center For the Seniors Housing & Care Industry (NIC) that the typical RC/AL resident is a woman with an average age of 85.7 years who is mobile, but needs assistance with two activities of daily living (ADLs). Males make up about 24.3 percent of the RC/AL resident population.

The same study revealed that the number of residents needing assistance varied considerably between types of assisted living facilities. Residents in RC/AL facilities typically need the most help with bathing (68 percent), and residents in dementia care facilities also require the most assistance with bathing (90 percent).

Assistance with medications is another service provided in RC/AL facilities. The 2006 survey (AAHSA et al. 2006) found that 86 percent of residents need some help managing their medications. State rules and regulations determine the training required of staff members who are permitted to assist with and/or administer medications. For example, in one state the medication aide must have one hour of training in medication assistance, in another state the aide must have eight hours of training, and in a third state only licensed nurses can administer medications to designated residents.

Resident Care Services

Assessment and Service Planning

The philosophy of RC/AL is integral to the assessment and planning of a resident's care. Each resident is treated with respect and dignity as the resident's total needs are assessed. The form used for assessment varies from facility to facility and from state to state. Nursing homes have a mandatory form for assessment (Minimum Data Set, or MDS forms), whereas RC/AL facilities do not.

In RC/AL facilities, the resident is fully involved in planning the services and care to be provided. Family members play an important role in the assessment process by providing information that the resident might not be able to provide. For example, when a resident is cognitively impaired, family members can provide valuable input. Primary consideration is given to the services that will promote the resident's independence and quality of life. Providing resident services that follow assessments is the basic reason RC/AL facilities exist. Experienced administrators agree that ensuring quality of care for each resident is of major concern. The resident should be fully informed of the services available; however, each resident has the right to refuse any service. Resident rights are discussed later in this chapter.

A thorough examination includes an assessment of physical problems and psychosocial functional needs conducted by qualified healthcare professionals to determine if facility personnel have the training and resources to respond to a resident's needs. The assessment should be holistic, considering the whole person. Some state regulations require that the assessment and health history be completed within a specified time, and these regulations have expanded the assessment categories to include the following items:

Physical: Chronic diseases, recent disease episodes, hospitalizations, mobility problems including impaired balance and falls, allergies, communicable diseases, substance abuse (e.g., pain medications, alcohol), skin conditions, sensory impairments, nutritional status, dietary needs, and any treatments that are needed as a result of present conditions.

Psychosocial: Cognitive and behavioral status including dementia, Alzheimer's disease or Alzheimer-like disorders; behaviors such as agitation, antisocial conduct (e.g., inappropriate touching, disrobing), and wandering; ability to reside in the facility with no history of impaired psychosocial behaviors. Preferences for social activities may be included here or assessed separately.

Self-administration of medications: Self-administration depends on many factors that are noted in the preceding assessment categories. The resident's physical and cognitive abilities help determine if the resident can self-administer.

Ability to function: Of utmost importance is the assessment of how the person functions—what he or she can do within the limitations of the physical and psychosocial status. Assisting the person to be as independent as possible is key to the quality of life that RC/AL facilities promote.

Cultural and religious preferences: Part of the total assessment must include preferences for cultural and religious practices. Some religions do not allow medical treatment. People from different cultures who speak foreign languages may need an interpreter to make their wishes known. (Assisted Living Assessment Workgroup 2003)

The requirements for assessment of the resident are regulated by each state; administrators must know and apply these regulations (National Center for Assisted Living 2005). Policies that direct the total assessment process must be written and followed. Assessment should occur before admission or soon after. Some states do not require that assessment be performed before admission. Other professionals may be involved in the assessment, depending on the resident's condition and previous health history. Psychological (e.g., cognitive ability, memory) and social status (e.g., family and community relationships) information, physical and functional status (ability to perform activities of daily living [ADLs] and instrumental activities of

daily living [IADLs]) information, dietary requirements, and preferences for recreational and social activities are gathered about the resident. Included among independent activities is the resident's ability to self-administer medications. Medication assistance is frequently a need of residents and one of the reasons a person enters an RC/AL facility.

When the assessment is complete, the plan of care, often referred to as the **negotiated service agreement**, can be written. The administrator will have a plan individualized for the resident that includes the client's/resident's choices picked from a list of recommended services. The administrator is responsible for having the plan of care reviewed routinely and immediately after a change in the resident's condition. Any change in the resident's condition or preferences warrants a new assessment and a renewed or modified service agreement.

Personal Services

Each RC/AL facility has a specific population or populations for whom services are provided. It is fairly common to find a facility that serves the older adult population in a general setting and the cognitively impaired in a special care unit. After consulting state regulations, each owner and/or administrator must decide which services will be provided in a facility. Each state has its own regulations about the extent of services that can be offered. For example, states issue specific regulations and rules that govern the requirements for care to provide services for special populations such as those with cognitive impairment. In general, the services offered in RC/AL facilities are as follows:

- Three meals a day, usually in a common area
- Assistance with activities of daily living (ADLs), such as eating, bathing, dressing, toileting, and walking
- Transportation
- Housekeeping services
- Access to medical and health services

- Staff who respond to scheduled and unscheduled needs
- 24-hour security
- Emergency call system
- Exercise and wellness programs
- Medication management
- Personal laundry services
- Social and recreational activities
- Assistance with instrumental activities of daily living (IADLs)

It is reasonable to expect that residents who are growing older in a facility will have changing needs. The administrator may discover that new services are needed as the conditions of residents change. For example, different recreational activities or exercise programs may be needed to counter residents' declining ability to ambulate. Some RC/AL facilities have packaged services that come at a basic cost, and any additional services provided are at an additional cost. For example, assistance with ADLs is included in the basic package, but fees are added for mending laundry and providing transportation (Assisted Living Federation of America 2006). Some facilities are moving to an à la carte system in which residents pick and choose services. Some states have regulations that designate who cannot be in the RC/AL facility because the services they require are beyond what the staff can provide.

Enhanced Services and Levels of Care

Some facilities offer enhanced services that typically are priced separately and in addition to the basic monthly residential fees. Dementia care or care of those with cognitive impairment is an enhanced service when offered in addition to traditional services. Other enhanced services include hospice or end-of-life care, skilled nursing care, and therapies such as oxygen and respiratory therapy.

States apply more stringent rules to provision of these services. For example, some states permit facilities to provide skilled services for limited amounts of time if the facility is not licensed to provide skilled services. States have been encouraged to establish levels of care for enhanced services and standards that must be met in providing them (Center for Medicare Advocacy 2003). The administrator must know that if skilled services are provided, qualified healthcare professionals are needed to deliver them, which can result in increased costs to the facility and the residents. Medicare and Medicaid will pay for outside services, such as physical and occupational therapies, for eligible residents when residents' physicians prescribe them.

The RC/AL administrator must decide how additional types of therapy will be provided. Communities have a number of rehabilitation service agencies that work with RC/AL facilities and other long term care providers. The administrator can negotiate with outside providers to set up service contracts that will make available the best scope of services at the most reasonable costs. Contract negotiation is discussed further in chapter 7. On the other hand, depending on the number of residents who require additional services, it may be more economical to hire appropriate professionals to work in the facility.

It is important that the resident and family members are fully involved as much as possible in deciding on which enhanced services the resident requires and that these services are made available when needed. For example, a resident's admission assessment might reveal that the resident requires only basic monthly services; however, as the resident's condition and needs change, rehabilitation-type services might need to be added to the resident's service mix.

Medication Delivery, Pharmacy, and Medication Assistance

Each state has its own regulations about how residents continue to receive their medications when they enter RC/AL facilities. The resident has a right to choose the pharmacy; however, many RC/AL administrators make contractual arrangements with a specific pharmacy for delivery of medications. The

15

administrator must ensure that the facility has policies that direct how medications are delivered to residents.

Increasingly, pharmacists are important partners in the care of residents in RC/AL facilities. Pharmacists can assist residents in choosing an appropriate drug plan that Medicare authorizes through insurance companies; family members should also be contacted to assist the resident in selection of the best plan. The wise administrator ensures that the pharmacist is also involved in overseeing each resident's pharmaceutical regimen so that there are no drug interactions or duplications. The RC/AL facility's contract with the pharmacist should include provision of these services.

Many RC/AL residents are on multiple medications, and the new Medicare Part D prescription drug coverage (effective January 2006) requires RC/AL administrators to comply with a variety of complex regulations related to pharmaceuticals. Administrators must be knowledgeable about Medicare Part D and how it affects residents. Medicare pays a resident's insurance company for the partial cost of medications. The resident must contribute a co-payment for medications unless the person meets eligibility requirements for paying nothing.

About 86 percent of RC/AL residents require assistance with medications (AAHSA et al. 2006). Some people require only cues or reminders to take their medications, whereas others need help opening containers, reading labels, swallowing pills, and remembering to take medications. State regulations that govern medication assistance and identifying who can assist residents and/or administer medications vary. RC/AL facilities are increasing their use of unlicensed assistive personnel (UAPs) in assisting with medications. UAPs must have training in medication assistance and the limitations they have in helping with medications. Medication assistance requires following the *rights* of medication delivery to residents: the right medication, at the right time, in the right dose, to the right person, using the right route,

and documented in the right way. Medications taken by residents must be documented by the person assisting or administering them. In some states, medication assistance by UAPs is governed by the boards of nursing and the rules that these boards promulgate. The administrator must know these rules and apply them appropriately.

Medication assistance in RC/AL facilities is a major responsibility that has continued to cause problems for all concerned. Administrators face at least three major challenges concerning medication assistance (American Society of Consultant Pharmacists 2003). First, the frail elderly person in an RC/AL facility is subject to drug reactions, interactions, and changes in physical and mental status as a result of taking multiple medications. In addition, aging persons absorb and excrete drugs more slowly, and these factors may cause negative drug reactions. Elderly people must be monitored closely so that their medications do not cause these disturbances. Second, administrators face the challenge of a lack of professional oversight of medication assistance. Unlicensed medication assistants are not educated or licensed to monitor residents' regimens. Also, they may unknowingly violate the six rights of medication administration described earlier. Problems of lack of oversight that include administering the wrong medication to the wrong resident, medications left at the bedside, and medications emptied into the assistant's hand and then transferred to the hand of the resident, the latter of which violates dictates of infection control as well as medication assistance, have arisen (Witmer 2005). The third challenge is the safe storage and disposition of the drugs. When drugs are no longer needed, they must be destroyed properly.

To meet these challenges of medication assistance, the American Society of Consultant Pharmacists (2003) recommends the following for administrators:

- A structured medication system (including acquisition, storage, administration, and disposition of medications)

- Competent staff (employing qualified, educated staff, who are evaluated routinely for performing the tasks and duties according to policies and job description)
- A continuous quality improvement program (routinely monitoring the program for needed improvements)
- Accountability (meeting state standards for medication assistance)

Residents who can self-administer their medications are identified on admission to the RC/AL facility. It is important to clarify the policy for those who take their own medications and for all aspects of the medication system. Medication must be stored safely and away from other residents. State regulations vary on these policies as well.

Prescription abbreviations that are commonly used for medications are listed here:

a.c.	before meals
p.c.	after meals
h.s.	hour of sleep or bedtime
b.i.d.	twice daily
t.i.d.	three times a day
q.i.d.	four times a day
q4h	every four hours
p.r.n.	when necessary or as needed
p.o.	by mouth
gtt	drop
cap.	capsule
tab.	tablet

Food Services

Food and the way it is served can be among the most enjoyable pleasures people have in life. One facet of the American culture is that most social events revolve around food. Residents in RC/AL facilities are not much different from other Americans. They look forward to the dining service and the sociability that it allows. Administrators who focus on the resident provide menu choices at different hours.

The RC/AL administrator is responsible for ensuring that the facility food is of good quality, nourishing, and meets the needs and preferences of the people being served. The latest publicized USDA food pyramid called MyPyramid contains the food groups and suggested servings for eating a balanced diet and can be a good guide for planning nutritional food programs (U.S. Department of Agriculture 2005). The new MyPyramid was revised to recommend more specific dietary recommendations based on age, gender, and activity level. Generally, the old food pyramid recommended eating a range of food servings, such as 6 to 12 servings per day of grains, without identifying who should eat 6 servings and who should eat 12. The new MyPyramid takes a decidedly more individualized approach to nutritional needs.

Food service demands a lot of attention from the administrator. Planning, implementing, and evaluating how the nutritional needs of residents are met require a lot of time. RC/AL residents are long term and they, and at times their family members, may complain if the food service is not satisfactory.

The food service area influences the facility operations 24 hours a day (Allen 2004). In addition to the three meals that are usually served, late-night snacks for people who are up at night and food for celebrations and special events are served. Many RC/AL facilities provide snacks for residents in a pantry area around the clock. Food service is also dependent on other departments in the facility, such as the laundry department for linens and the maintenance department for keeping the kitchen in good operating order.

The administrator is responsible for ensuring a qualified individual, registered dietician or dietary consultant, oversees the preparation of nutritional diets and any special diets required to meet resident needs. Some facilities have a dietician on staff. Other administrators consult with qualified dieticians. Functions performed by personnel in the food service department are as follows:

- Ensuring tasty and nutritional food is prepared and served at the correct temperature

- Consulting on nutritional assessments of residents
- Overseeing/consulting about residents' weight gains and losses
- Recommending/providing food substitutes as requested
- Catering for facility functions
- Maintaining the cleanliness of the kitchen and dining areas
- Handling and storing dry foods and refrigerated foods properly
- Training and maintaining healthy condition of staff
- Dishwashing
- Disposing garbage and refuse; caring for hazardous materials (e.g., detergents, insecticides) (Allen 2004)

The RC/AL administrator must know local and state regulations that apply to the food service department. Other nongovernmental organizations that provide guidelines for healthy meals include the American Diabetes Association and American Dietetic Association.

In meeting the needs of residents, therapeutic diets may be required. A therapeutic diet is one that is ordered by a physician and considered part of the treatment for a condition (e.g., difficulty chewing) or disease/disorder (e.g., diabetes, stomach ulcer). Other diets are fairly common: low sodium, low fat, high protein, high fiber, and mechanical soft, which means the food is softened or only soft foods are served.

The nutritional assessment on admission should include the person's nutritional status and ability to eat independently. Assistive devices must be available to help people with certain disabilities eat independently. For example, a person with arthritic changes in his or her hands may need eating utensils with enlarged handles. Some people may need help in preparing to eat food (e.g., opening containers, cutting meat). Staff must be available to help these individuals whether residents choose to eat in their room or in the dining room.

Some facilities may offer different dining rooms or one large dining area where people are assigned seating. Some facilities offer menus from which residents can make choices. Preferences must be honored if the resident does not agree with the seating arrangements or is unhappy with the food. Ideally, the resident makes the choice of what to eat from a menu and decides where to sit to eat.

To evaluate the food service, the administrator should eat in the dining area to experience firsthand the quality of the food and service. Talking with residents and conducting periodic surveys also help the administrator stay on top of any potential problems.

Depending on the size of the facility, food services may be performed by in-house employees or outsourced to a catering service. Regardless of how food service is provided, it is always a concern because of the many meals prepared, the preferences of the people being served, and the potential danger of contamination if the standards for safety, cleanliness, and food storage are not maintained. In addition, staff must be healthy, free of any disease, and trained to follow food service standards.

Activity Services

Residents have different preferences for activities offered inside and outside the facility. Activities many times serve a therapeutic purpose. For example, a person with arthritis in the hands should exercise the hands in different ways, such as by making crafts, to keep the fingers from contracting into positions that limit their use. Activities also provide socialization and enjoyment that enhances quality of life. Health and wellness programs add information and exercises that are geared to improving individual health. Outside activities help residents keep connected to the community and reduce their feelings of isolation.

Activities for persons who are cognitively impaired must be planned with care. The Alzheimer's Association recommends activities that are geared to the cognitive level of each person and offered in a calm environment. Activities that are recommended are short—no longer than 30 minutes—and meaningful, with the purpose of keeping individuals as independent as possible. Selection of activities depends on the abilities of each person. Suggestions include gardening, word games, intergenerational projects, musical programs, and making decorations. For some individuals, these activities may be conducted on a one-to-one basis, whereas other individuals may do well in a small group. Staff must be thoroughly trained in how to approach persons with cognitive impairment.

There is a trend in some residences to follow the Eden Alternative fostered by a physician named Dr. William Thomas. Dr. Thomas's philosophy of helping people grow in nursing homes by bringing in pets, flowers (gardening), birds, and children forged a revolutionizing alternative. This idea is frequently referred to as culture change and has spread to many RC/AL residences across the country. Residents become involved in the activities that have to do with the pets, birds, gardening, and children. Dr. Thomas's efforts have brought lonely, withdrawn people back to a "life worth living" (Thomas 2004).

Housekeeping Services

Keeping the facility clean with a home-like appearance is the job of the housekeeping personnel. Housekeeping staff members contribute to the safety, sanitation, and pleasant look of the facility as a whole and the living spaces of each resident. Infection control should be part of the training of housekeeping personnel. Personnel must know about disease prevention and disease transmission and must practice measures to keep the environment as clean as possible. The specific duties of housekeeping personnel and maintenance personnel must be clarified because at times their duties seem to conflict. For example, who cleans up after maintenance personnel create debris during a repair? The logical answer is the maintenance people who created the debris.

The size of the RC/AL facility determines how many staff members are required to keep the facility clean. In a large facility, housekeeping is a department. Cleaning for residents may be scheduled once a week and at other times when needed. In small facilities with few people, light housekeeping is usually done every day with heavier cleaning once a week. Housekeeping for residents normally includes at no extra charge cleaning bathrooms, emptying trash, dusting furniture, vacuuming carpets, and/or mopping floors and changing linens. The facility may charge additional fees for cleaning kitchens/kitchenettes, windows, and any other item not included in the original agreement. In some facilities, residents clean their own rooms and rooms of others in exchange for money. This arrangement must be in writing and signed by both the resident and the administrator.

Cleaning the facility spaces includes cleaning the walls, drapes, and furniture in public areas. Routines are usually established for what will be cleaned at what time. A clean and pleasant facility is a primary concern of persons considering a move to an RC/AL facility.

Housekeeping personnel must be trained in keeping their work areas safe and their cleaning supplies away from residents. Controls must be in place for how cleaning materials are handled. Signs warning people of wet areas should always be visible. The person in charge should have a routine of checking areas used by residents to be sure the standards for housekeeping are maintained and improved when necessary.

Laundry Services

Laundry services are a concern of residents and are usually basic services offered by RC/AL facilities. In smaller facilities, laundry may be done in-house. In larger facilities, it may be contracted to an outside source. Some residents may prefer to do their own laundry in machines that are conveniently available, or their family members do their laundry. Resident want clean clothes and usually want their favorite clothes available for wearing. Most facilities advise residents to mark their clothing clearly to avoid loss and/or laundry returned to the wrong person.

The administrator who chooses to do laundry on the premises must have a staff member in charge to supervise and train laundry personnel about the following duties:

- Separation of dirty laundry from clean laundry
- Proper precautions for handling dirty linens and clothing; wearing of gloves for protection from body fluids; cleaning and protecting areas where dirty laundry is placed before washing
- Collection, mending, sorting, washing, drying, and returning laundry to the right person (laundry should have some mark/name indicating to whom it belongs)
- Cleaning of equipment and maintaining of equipment (with help of the maintenance department)
- Possible assistance of residents who wish to do their own laundry

In addition to the basic laundry services fee, some facilities may charge additional fees for some of the preceding duties. The person in charge of the laundry should periodically monitor workers and the work areas as well as interview residents to ensure services are satisfactory.

Transportation Services

Family members play an active role in transporting their loved ones; however, they are not always available, so transportation services in an RC/AL facility are invaluable. The RC/AL facility should have some form of available transportation or be willing to make arrangements for transportation. The average 85-year-old woman who represents the typical resident is not likely to be driving her own car unless she is still very independent. Transportation services allow her and others to continue to participate in activities in the community.

Some facility owners purchase a van that is wheelchair accessible. The name of the facility is painted on the side of the vehicle, a good form of advertising. The van or another roomy vehicle is used to transport residents to appointments, shopping, and social activities. Transportation services add to the quality of life and increase opportunities for people to continue activities independently once they arrive at their destinations. Usually, facilities have a rule that residents must sign out and in when they leave and return to the facility as a way of keeping track of residents, especially if any persons have cognitive impairments.

Some administrators find alternatives to buying a vehicle. Leasing a vehicle, contractual agreements with an outside transportation agency, and coupons for taxi services are other ways of providing transportation to residents without purchasing vehicles. The administrator must weigh the costs and benefits of leasing. In some communities, taxi companies offer books of coupons for seniors that are much less expensive to use than regular taxi services. A main concern for transportation alternatives is accessibility for persons with disabilities. Administrators must also adhere to any state regulations regarding transportation services in RC/AL facilities.

Other Healthcare Services and Resources

RC/AL facilities are not meant to be all things to residents. The administrator should be knowledgeable about healthcare services not available at the facility that are offered in the community. Home health agencies provide care to residents in RC/AL facilities. Other agencies provide rehabilitation services such as physical, occupational, and speech therapy. Massage is another popular therapy usually available in the community. Health and wellness sessions are an excellent addition to facilities. A list of community resources and service costs should be made available to residents and potential residents who may be coming from another state.

Community resources should also be available to residents and their families. Maintaining connections by continuing to participate in activities in the community provides for residents' continued enjoyment and quality of life. Residents' choices of activities will vary. Having information on community resources at their fingertips helps them to decide which to participate in. Senior centers provide many activities as do educational institutions, churches, and specialized community groups, such as garden clubs. Local senior publications seem to be on the rise. Making these publications available to residents gives them another resource they can use to find out about activities offered locally.

Some residents may want to volunteer in community organizations or within the facility. Facility policies should be established on how and where residents can volunteer. Volunteers who supplement the staff need training, and providing training should be part of the policy. Volunteering helps residents to feel valued and needed, both of which are important to self-esteem.

Professional Ethics and Resident Care

The Merriam-Webster dictionary defines *ethics* as a code of morals that relate to conduct. In RC/AL facilities, an ethical code of conduct revolves around what is right and best for the resident. The administrator should consider two major areas of emphasis on how ethics is applied in the RC/AL facility: (1) conduct of the staff, and (2) decisions about and for the resident.

Conduct of the Staff

The administrator and each staff member must conduct themselves appropriately at all times. Respect and dignity are shown to residents and other staff and to all persons with whom they come in contact. Professional groups usually have a written code of ethics specific to their discipline. For example, physicians and professional nurses have their own ethical codes of conduct. The administrator should establish a code of conduct for facility personnel that includes the behaviors expected on the job.

Decisions about and for the Resident

There are times when ethical decisions must be made about the care of a resident. Family members may have a difficult time deciding what should happen in the care of their loved one. The administrator should have an ethics committee composed of knowledgeable representatives from various community groups. The committee might include a physician, home health nurse, hospice provider, ethical expert, and a facility staff member. The purpose of the ethics committee is to consider the options for care and to offer recommendations to the decision makers. An ethics committee may become involved in situations when no advance directive is available for a resident and the family is trying to make a decision about whether to continue treatment. The ethics committee provides support for the staff as well. The committee may also become involved in resident rights issues when ethics is involved (e.g., resident abuse).

The American College of Health Care Administrators (ACHCA) has a code of ethics that applies to administrators of long term care facilities. Administrators are advised to visit the ACHCA Web site to view the entire code. The code of ethics is briefly outlined here:

- Expectation I: Individuals shall hold paramount the welfare of persons for whom care is provided.
- Expectation II: Individuals shall maintain high standards of professional conduct.

Paramount (최우선으로 하다)

- Expectation III: Individuals shall strive, in all matters relating to their professional functions, to maintain a professional posture that places <u>paramount</u> the interests of the facility and its residents.
- Expectation IV: Individuals shall honor their responsibilities to the public, their profession, and their relationships with colleagues and members of related professions. (ACHCA 2004)

Recordkeeping Systems

RC/AL administrators must keep records and other required documentation that <u>pertain to resident care</u>. Regulations are different from state to state, but some recordkeeping rules are similar. <mark>Before starting a record</mark> for a resident, the administrator should be certain <mark>the facility is right for the new resident</mark>, that <mark>services are available to meet resident needs and preferences, and that the decision has been made for the resident to enter the facility. The following resident records are usually required:</mark>

- <mark>Information identifying</mark> the resident: name; previous address; date of birth; gender; date of admission; religious preference/affiliation; physician's name, telephone number, and address; name of legally responsible persons, their telephone numbers and addresses; family contacts; and emergency telephone numbers and addresses
- <mark>Assessments</mark>, such as health history and complete physical with mental, psychosocial, and functional assessments, and medical records
- <mark>Individualized service plan</mark>
- <mark>Special nutritional</mark>/dietary requirements
- <mark>Pharmacy</mark> requirements regarding purchasing and dispensing of medications and ability of resident to self-administer or need for assistance
- <mark>Written need</mark> and specific arrangements for skilled care as appropriate

- Resident agreement <u>delineating</u> policies, standards, resident rights, and responsibilities
- Written complaints and investigation of mental or physical abuse and follow-up according to state requirements
- Written and signed risk agreements
- End of life preferences

The following records may or may not be required but are recommended:

- Fire and evacuation procedures and dates drills were performed
- Logs of incidents that may or may not <u>pertain to</u> resident incidents
- Staff records that include names, addresses, telephone numbers, medical exams, testing for tuberculosis, vaccines (e.g., flu), background checks, licenses, certificates, continuing education sessions and training, hours worked, awards
- Copies of facility licenses and inspections
- Written proof of heating, ventilation, and air conditioning inspections
- Contracts with outside vendors
- Policy and procedures of services provided and other documents required by the state

All records must be stored in safe places that ensure their protection and confidentiality. Resident records must be stored according to the requirements of the <u>Health Insurance Portability and Accountability Act</u> of <u>1996, known as HIPAA</u>. Two issues that apply to resident records are privacy and security. HIPAA establishes security standards to protect access to protected health information by requiring passwords for the electronic (computerized) storage and transmission of information. HIPAA also requires that all healthcare facilities, including RC/AL facilities, develop a Notice of Privacy Practices that must be distributed to all residents. The administrator must be familiar with and implement these practices, some of which are listed as follows, as they apply to RC/AL facilities. The conditions for these practices must also be made known to residents. Administrators must comply with other practices besides the ones listed here.

- The designation of a privacy officer who oversees the resident's requests
- A resident's right to view and to request a copy of his or her medical record
- A resident's right to request a change in the medical record
- A resident's right to request restriction of use of his or her information as long as the restriction does not interfere with treatment, payment, or operations

The administrator must be alert to the practices of the facility that protect residents' privacy. This means avoiding dining room, elevator, and hallway discussions that involve protected resident information and following the "minimum necessary rule" when responding to telephone calls or other requests for information about particular residents. The minimum necessary rule basically requires that healthcare personnel use only the minimum amount of information to get the job done. For example, when ordering a wheelchair, the resident's height and weight may be necessary information but not the resident's diagnosis. This rule applies to all forms of communication (e-mail, fax, etc.). Staff members must know to maintain confidentiality at all times, and that means conversing about residents only with people who have the right to know.

Move-In and Move-Out Issues

Move In

People who enter RC/AL facilities come from a variety of settings. About 60 percent come from their own homes or an apartment except for those in freestanding dementia care who move from a family residence (lived with adult children or other relatives) more than 50 percent of the time (AAHSA et al. 2006). Approximately 16 percent relocate from a combination assisted living/independent living facility, and 24 percent relocate

from a continuing care retirement residence. Another 15 percent relocate to assisted living from a combination assisted living and nursing home facility. Approximately 40 percent of assisted living residents move into an assisted living community immediately following release from an acute care hospital, rehabilitation hospital, or short-stay nursing facility (AAHSA et al. 2006). These people need assistance of some kind.

Many RC/AL residents hope to return to their former lives and are anxious about their new living arrangements. Every person entering a new place to live has different emotional reactions. Relocation is hard on older adults. Research has shown that with each move, the aging individual with compromised or failing health experiences increased stress that may affect his or her behavior and health status (Linton and Lach 2006). Newly admitted individuals need empathy, a warm reception, and close observation. This is especially true of people who are cognitively impaired. They need a quiet, calm environment with a limited number of caregivers who are trained in the expected and unexpected behaviors that may be exacerbated by the change in environment.

From a marketing and hospitality perspective, the administrator should be sure potential residents meet the admission criteria and should have a plan to help each person gradually adjust to the idea of relocating to an RC/AL residence. Getting to know the individual and his or her family as much as possible and providing opportunities for the person and family members to get to know more about the facility, including activities offered, routines, and the staff who will be looking after the person, are good first steps. Interviews with the potential resident and the family and tours of the facility should be conducted soon after admission. Administrators can invite potential residents to visit the facility during a social event as another way to help reassure the person that the move will be a good one. It is recommended that potential residents have contact with one facility person skilled in meeting and greeting new people. This staff person should be available to potential residents to answer questions and provide any additional information upon request.

Once a person is admitted, that person's every request and preference should be acknowledged and honored as much as possible Caring staff who are informed of the person's health status and needs should provide close observation and frequent communication with the new resident. Admission documentation is discussed later in this chapter.

Move Out

Of persons who move out of RC/AL facilities, about 33.5 percent move to a nursing home; 30.2 percent expire; 6.7 percent move to another RC/AL facility; 6.6 percent go home; 4.4 percent move to a relative's home; 4.2 percent move to a hospital; and 6.5 percent move somewhere not determined (AAHSA et al. 2006). It is very important for personnel in RC/AL facilities to assist residents and their families with whatever care and other arrangements are needed. Communication, orally and in written form, with other receiving entities about the needs of the person leaving is crucial for continuity of care. Examples of how this collaboration with receiving facilities and/or entities is accomplished are listed here:

- Move to a hospital: Oral and written reports of the person's diagnoses and changes that occurred, including physical, psychosocial, and functional. An RC/AL staff person should visit the hospital to help answer any questions or concerns the resident and family have, and to plan for the resident's return to the RC/AL facility if appropriate.
- Move to a nursing facility: Oral and written report of the person's history at the RC/AL facility, including the reasons for the transfer to the nursing facility. An RC/AL staff person should visit the nursing facility to help answer any questions or concerns the resident and family have,

and to plan for the resident's return to the RC/AL facility if appropriate.
- Move to another RC/AL facility: Oral and written report of the person's history, including the reasons for transfer to another RC/AL facility. It may not be advisable for RC/AL staff member to visit the resident in another facility if the situation is not friendly.
- Move to home: Coordination of services, such as rehabilitation services, that must continue in the home. Arrangements for services should be made before the resident leaves the RC/AL facility. An RC/AL staff person should visit the home to ensure services are being provided. The RC/AL facility has no responsibility to provide services or arrange for services once the resident is discharged from the facility.
- Move if the person expires: Assist the family with funeral arrangements.

The administrator can also ease the stress of transition of residents to other destinations by providing assistance with the move. States set requirements for moves that administrators must follow. When possible, the administrator should make a follow-up call and/or send a letter to the former resident and family expressing appreciation for their spending time in the facility and a wish that they are doing well, or offering condolences in case of a death.

Resident Care Policies and Procedures

Resident care policies and procedures establish the standards that must be met in the RC/AL facility. They are written to meet the requirements of state and local laws, as well as federal regulations (Center for Medicare Advocacy 2003). The administrator must be alert for changes in state regulations that may prompt changes in facility policies.

Policies may be written for other reasons. For example, an incident may occur for which no policy was written. So that employees know how to respond if a similar incident happens, a policy and set of procedures must be written. *Policies* provide the general direction for activities that are performed by RC/AL staff. *Procedures* are the specific steps to be taken in carrying out the policy. When facilities have policies and procedures, employees know ahead of time what is expected of them. Policies and procedures for each of the service areas and for other activities that relate to contacts with residents and the public must exist.

Admission Policies

The kind of services offered by the facility are those allowed by state regulation. The admission policy and procedures include the type of services offered. The resident agreement that is part of the admission policy indicates which services meet the needs and preferences of the resident. The resident agreement usually stipulates which services are not allowed. The resident agreement also includes costs of services, responsibilities of the resident and family as appropriate, responsibilities of the RC/AL facility staff, and any other general provisions. Some facilities ask residents to create a list of possessions they are bringing to the facility.

At this time, it is important for the administrator to clarify the resident's wishes regarding **advance directives, do not resuscitate orders (DNR),** and preferred funeral arrangements. If the resident has an advance directive and DNR order that state his or her wishes about end-of-life care, it is not necessary to have a physician's order to prevent resuscitation if the resident has a cardiac arrest.

Advance directives also include a **living will** and a legal **power of attorney** for healthcare. A living will is a document that contains the resident's wishes about treatment and life-sustaining measures. The person who is the resident's power of attorney (POA) for

healthcare is a person designated by the resident to make decisions regarding the resident's healthcare when the resident is deemed incapable of making his or her own decisions. States have regulations that stipulate how a person is determined to be incapable of decision making.

Admission is also a good time for the administrator to learn if the resident has a **guardian** or **conservator.** In general, states define these roles in the following way: a guardian has legal authority to act on behalf of, and make decisions for, the resident. The guardian's basic duty is to provide for the personal care and maintenance of the incapacitated person. The guardian is appointed by the court to make decisions for the resident if the resident is determined to be incompetent.

A conservator is a person who is appointed by a court of law to manage the estate of a protected person. A conservator's authority relates to the management of assets and property, rather than the personal care of the resident.

Admission policies and procedures should address the issues of care mentioned here. For example, a resident may feel that no advance directive are necessary, but the administrator must be alert to what the resident may need in the future.

Resident Assessment Policies

State regulations specify what is to be included in the initial resident assessment and may state within what time period the assessment should be completed. Residents should be reassessed when any changes in their condition occur. Policies for assessment and reassessment must reflect state requirements. The initial assessment includes the items described previously in the section titled "Assessment and Service Planning." Reasons and timing of reassessments should be specified in the policy. Some states require routine reassessments to be sure all needs of residents are being met. It is the administrator's responsibility to follow up on residents, even though the responsibility for reassessment might be delegated to a licensed nurse or other staff member. The administrator should have background knowledge about physical, psychosocial, and functional changes that can be expected in aging people so that they can anticipate changes and respond to them.

Personal Care Policies

Personal care policies are based on the personal care services included in the negotiated service agreements. Policies should state how services are provided. For example, the policies specify that internal staff provide some personal care services and/or some services are contracted with outside agencies (e.g., physical therapy). Policies must comply with state regulations.

Medication Management Policies

Policies for how medication is administered or medication assistance is provided must be clarified. Policies should reflect state requirements and how the facility staff complies with those requirements. Medication management policies should include resident self-administration rules, type of assistance trained staff members will provide, and policies on storage of medications.

Dietary/Food Service Management Policies

Dietary/food service policies specify who is in charge of the food service/dietary department, meal planning, dietary preparation (qualified specialist), food purchases, dining arrangements, and food storage and sanitation. Training of food service personnel also should be included in the policies. Policies must comply with state and local regulations.

Activity Policies

Activity policies should be based on the state regulations that usually serve as guides for the types of activities RC/AL facilities offer. Activities should be available for residents whose functional ability ranges from independent to low level, and from one-on-one to groups.

Housekeeping Policies

Housekeeping policies focus on guidelines for providing a clean and attractive, home-like environment for residents. Policies specify the frequency of cleaning resident and public spaces. Procedures should include how hazardous cleaning materials are kept out of reach of residents. Infection control measures should be part of the training included in the policies.

Laundry Policies

Laundry policies include how laundry services are provided for residents and the facility. Procedures are necessary for maintaining a clean laundry environment and protection of the staff when handling dirty laundry.

Maintenance Policies

Maintenance policies and procedures include a schedule of maintenance services and routines for keeping equipment throughout the facility in good running order.

Infection Control

In any service related to healthcare, infection control is extremely important. Many people come in contact with each other, and each person brings a different set of defenses against illness and infections. RC/AL facilities are conducive to the spread of illness, especially communicable diseases, such as common colds, influenza (flu), and dysentery, unless precautions are in place to prevent spread of infection. The purpose of an infection control plan is to provide and maintain a safe, sanitary, and comfortable environment free of disease and infection.

State regulations dictate the infection control measures that must be in place in an RC/AL facility. The administrator should develop an infection control program for any possible infection or disease that might occur. Consultation with representatives from the Centers for Disease Control and Prevention (CDC) and the Occupational Safety and Health Administration (OSHA) can be extremely helpful. Some components of an effective infection control program are listed here.

For Residents

- Early identification of residents with low immune systems (e.g., frail elderly, persons with HIV/AIDS, persons with pressure sores)
- Early detection of a resident with any skin, eye, respiratory, or gastrointestinal infection
- Procedures for isolating infected resident(s) to prevent spread
- Vaccination of residents against pneumonia and influenza
- Policies regarding transfer of residents as needed
- Screening for TB as a prerequisite for admission

For Staff

- Medical examinations and testing to ensure staff are healthy and free of disease before working and after exposure to infected resident(s)
- Training for frequent handwashing using proper techniques
- Training in isolation techniques and avoidance of cross-contamination as appropriate
- Training in use of standard precautions regarding body fluids
- Work restrictions for ill employees and vaccinations to prevent illnesses
- Orientation of all personnel in infection control standards and routine updates on regulations

For Facility

- A surveillance plan for early detection of circumstances that produce infection and disease; investigation of nosocomial (facility-based) and community-acquired infections
- Proper use of disinfectants, antiseptics, and so forth in accordance with Environmental Protection Agency (EPA) standards and Food and Drug Administration (FDA) labels
- Sanitation of all equipment that is used for residents (e.g., tubs, whirlpools)
- Prompt attention to any indication of a communicable illness in an RC/AL facility; administrators must know the local reporting laws and the state's requirements

Emergency Preparedness

Emergencies happen even though a facility is well managed. An RC/AL administrator can prepare for some emergencies that are more likely to occur in the geographical area in which the facility is located. Policies and procedures and a plan for how to evacuate the facility should be written in preparation for potential disasters. The policies, procedures, and plans should be reviewed at least annually. Some RC/AL administrators conduct an annual drill to simulate how to evacuate residents and staff in case of an emergency. The following list contains emergency situations that require a plan.

- Bioterrorism attacks
- Severe weather, such as hurricanes and tornadoes
- Bomb threats
- Floods
- Earthquakes
- Violence from inside or outside the facility

Many of these situations will involve evacuation. In some cases, such as severe flooding that results from bad weather, an evacuation plan must be implemented. Evacuation requires arrangements for the residents to move to another location. Preparedness requires having contracts in place for resident transportation services, as well as with another RC/AL facility or healthcare provider that will accept the residents. Depending on circumstances, the evacuation of residents may mean the receiving facility is in another state. Hurricane Katrina taught RC/AL administrators a number of lessons about how quickly and how far residents must go to safety. It is advisable to learn about the local area's plan for disaster, and ask if it includes your residents. In a community disaster, the administrator must know who will conduct the evacuation to avoid conflicts with another facility that needs evacuation. Contracts should provide for the continuation of the following services:

- Lodging
- Food and water
- Pharmacy
- Transportation
- Linen service
- Health/medical services and equipment

Having access to resident records and advance directives becomes important in these kinds of emergencies. An emergency system for availability of records should be included in the emergency preparations. Critical resident information could be summarized into a set of records that is easily attainable, portable, and HIPAA compliant.

Emergency preparedness also includes training the personal care staff and others in first aid, cardiopulmonary resuscitation (CPR), and the Heimlich maneuver to relieve choking. Retraining should be on an annual basis and updated as changes are needed. A plan must be in place for other emergencies such as heart attacks and accidents. Staff must be informed of the procedures to follow in these cases. Accidents must be thoroughly investigated and preventive measures applied whenever possible. Accidents should be

referred to the quality assurance committee for problem solving.

Resident Rights and Responsibilities

Key to providing services to residents is the protection of resident rights. Resident rights may be different in different states. Recognizing that these rights underlie the autonomy of residents and their decision-making power, the National Center for Assisted Living (2006) advocates that residents' rights include the following:

- To privacy
- To be treated at all times with dignity and respect
- To control personal finances
- To retain and have use of personal possessions
- To interact freely with others in the assisted living residence and in the community
- To have freedom of religion
- To control receipt of health-related services
- To organize resident councils

Resident rights must be made known to the resident and family members on admission. States may have a set of rights that must be honored in the facility. Staff members must know and protect these rights in the delivery of care. The administrator should ensure that staff members are trained in the application of rights and that these rights are not violated. For example, when a resident refuses care and/or treatment, staff must recognize this as the resident's right. Staff members must know how to respond and follow the facility policy that protects the resident.

State regulations may also specify which types of rights violations must be reported. Mandatory reporting often includes situations of abuse, neglect, misappropriation of funds, accidents, and incidents of serious nature.

Negotiated Risk

An RC/AL resident may put him- or herself at risk (possible harm) for deteriorating health by refusing care or treatment. The administrator can expect that this kind of situation may occur; therefore, a policy of risk negotiation should be considered. A **negotiated risk agreement** allows the resident the right to make an independent decision about care with full knowledge of the risk involved. The resident and the RC/AL facility administrator sign the agreement. Concerns arise when a person with cognitive impairment makes a decision that involves risk. Family members and other concerned parties, such as a guardian, a person with power of attorney for healthcare, and possibly lawyers, become involved. Risk management is another topic that residents, families, and staff should know and understand.

Quality Assurance

Administrators use a quality assurance committee to ensure that all services provided to residents are of high quality, and that all departments are conducting activities according to standards. Quality assurance committees are composed of staff members who meet to review the activities of each department. They use an audit tool as a baseline for comparing standards compliance. This committee might also review any problems that occur and, after reviewing the facts and possible solutions, make recommendations for resolution of the problems.

Some RC/AL facilities employ an external compliance specialist to conduct an audit of the services offered and operations of the facility. Regardless of how quality assurance is conducted, it is one method the administrator can use to gauge the quality of services. Quality assurance is an ongoing activity that must also meet state regulations.

Dying and Death Issues

The RC/AL administrator has reasons to become involved in at least four issues surrounding dying and death.

1. The advance directives of a dying resident must be honored. Advance directives may include information specifying where the person wants to be at the time of death as well as the type and extent of care to be provided. The resident may want to leave the facility to die.
2. Administrators tend to want RC/AL residents to stay as long as possible. State regulations specify the conditions under which the resident can and cannot stay in an RC/AL facility, especially if a higher level of care that is beyond the services of the facility is required.
3. Hospice care is care of a dying person who a healthcare provider has predicted will pass away within a six-month period of time. Hospice care involves direct care of the person based on a comprehensive assessment from an interdisciplinary healthcare team that may include RC/AL staff or care provided by a contracted outside hospice service provider. Family counseling and bereavement services are included.

   Hospice care is a Medicare benefit. Medicare pays for hospice to qualified agencies that meet the required conditions of participation. Administrators must ensure the facility complies with state regulations when providing hospice care.
4. Administrators must understand the grieving process that residents and their family members, as well as staff members who care for the resident, may experience when a resident nears the end of life. The recognized stages of grief may cause the resident to withdraw and family members to express anger that is misdirected. The grieving process

29

includes stages of denial, anger, bargaining, acceptance, and depression. People may not experience the stages in order and often fluctuate between stages. When administrators can recognize the reactions to grieving, they can be better prepared to interact appropriately with residents, family members, and staff. Administrators must also recognize that staff members who become attached to residents experience varying degrees of grief when the resident dies and need some way to express their emotions. Administrators can make support groups for caregivers available in the facility.

RC/AL administrators face many challenges in managing quality resident care. The challenges begin when they admit residents to the facility and continue when providing services to meet resident needs and preferences in compliance with state regulations. Administrators are responsible for planning, implementing and evaluating facility services.

GLOSSARY

Advance directive: A statement executed by a person while of sound mind as to that person's wishes about the use of medical interventions for him or herself in case of the loss of his or her own decision-making capacity.

Conservator: A person who has the legal authority and duty to protect the assets of another, "protected person" (a minor or incompetent). A conservator is appointed by a court, in the same way that a guardian is appointed, but can only make decisions about property, not about medical care or other decisions personal to the protected person.

Do not resuscitate (DNR) order: An order by the physician, with respect to a specific patient, to the effect that, should cardiac arrest or respiratory arrest occur, no attempt should be made to give cardiopulmonary resuscitation to the patient.

Durable power of attorney: A power of attorney that remains (or becomes) effective when the principal becomes incompetent to act for himself or herself. (It should be noted that in most states, even an agent with a durable power of attorney cannot make medical treatment decisions for an incompetent patient, unless state law provides that he or she can or a court has given him or her specific authority.)

Guardian: A person who has the legal responsibility, and the authority to make decisions, for an incompetent person or a minor. A guardian is appointed by a court. The written guardianship order specifically states the authority of the guardian, and might convey authority to make decisions only about money and property management, or authority to make personal decisions (such as those regarding health care), or might convey authority to make both kinds of decisions.

Living will: A will concerning the life of the person executing the will, in which the individual provides guidance for circumstances under which they wish to refuse, or discontinue the use of, life-support measures administered to themselves should they become incompetent. (A living will is in contrast with the usual "last will and testament" in which the subject matter is the disposition of property or custody of minor children.)

Power of attorney: A written agreement under which one person (the "principal") authorizes another (the "agent") to act on his or her behalf. The agent need not be a lawyer. An ordinary power of attorney automatically terminates if the principal becomes incompetent. (See durable power of attorney.)

PRACTICE QUESTIONS

Read each of the following items carefully, and then select the best response.

1. When considering the admission of a resident, the RC/AL administrator must include which of the following factors in the admission decision?
   A. Cultural and religious preferences
   B. Disabilities of the resident
   C. All needs and preferences of the resident
   D. Family members assessed needs of the resident

   A B C D
   O O O O

2. Payment for assisted living services comes mostly from which source?
   A. Private pay
   B. Medicare
   C. Medicaid
   D. Social Security Income

   A B C D
   O O O O

3. Mrs. M. needs assistance with medications. This means her medications are best stored where?
   A. In her bedside table available to the assisting person
   B. In a locked compartment available to the assisting person
   C. In the office of the facility
   D. In the kitchen for distribution at meals

   A B C D
   O O O O

4. HIPAA is a federal act that mandates that each resident has the right to:
   A. be seen by their physician of choice.
   B. receive signed copies of Resident Rights and Grievance Procedures.
   C. take his/her medications on vacation
   D. privacy, security, and confidentiality of his/her records.

   A B C D
   O O O O

5. The risk agreement helps to clarify in writing the desire and right of:
   A. the resident to behave in ways that may be harmful and that the resident claims responsibility for the behavior
   B. the staff to assist with the resident's negative behavior and the staff's responsibility in doing so
   C. family members to assist with the resident's negative behavior
   D. the administrator to help the resident avoid negative behavior

   A B C D
   O O O O

6. Advance directives provide written instructions for end-of-life care. Which of the following statements names these documents?
   A. Guardianship
   B. Conservatorship
   C. Living will and power of attorney for healthcare
   D. Hospice contract and Durable Power of Attorney

   A B C D
   O O O O

7. Mr. Smith is admitted with a left-sided stroke and expects to be going home after several weeks of physical therapy (PT). In the meantime, his wife of 40 years dies at home. Mr. Smith refuses his PT therapy and wants to stay in his room. His behaviors are most likely caused by which of the following:
   A. Schizophrenia
   B. A second stroke
   C. Organic brain syndrome
   D. Depression

   A B C D
   ○ ○ ○ ○

8. Mrs. Jones just returned to the facility from the hospital after suffering from pneumonia. The caregiver notices that Mrs. Jones is disoriented, pulling at the bed linens, and feels very warm. Mrs. Jones's temperature is 102 degrees. The caregiver should report this immediately because Mrs. Jones is most likely in a state of:
   A. Relapse of pneumonia
   B. Delirium
   C. Recovery from pneumonia
   D. Hydration

   A B C D
   ○ ○ ○ ○

9. Internal and external activities should be part of the services offered to aging adults because theorists claim and residents say which of the following statements?
   A. Activities are expensive and they keep people from getting bored.
   B. Activities are good but hard for some people with disabilities.
   C. Activities help people stay connected with their previous lives.
   D. Activities help to distract people from their disabilities.

   A B C D
   ○ ○ ○ ○

10. It has been raining for almost a week. Your community has been alerted that the nearby river is about to crest, and heavy flooding of the lower land areas is a strong possibility. Your facility and several others are located in the flat land along the river. Your first action should be which of the following?
    A. Continue to monitor water level.
    B. Notify the residents they must vacate.
    C. Put the emergency plan into action.
    D. Pull the alarm for disaster warning.

    A B C D
    ○ ○ ○ ○

ANSWERS AND EXPLANATIONS

1. **Correct answer = C.** Cultural and religious preferences and disabilities should be considered, but assessment of the resident should not be limited by these preferences. Families should be consulted; however, the focus is on the comprehensive range of needs of the resident.

2. **Correct answer = A.** Medicare does not pay for RC/AL. Private pay is by far the greatest source of payment. States can apply for Medicaid waivers that help to pay part of the costs of RC/AL. Persons on Social Security Income may also receive some financial assistance.

3. **Correct answer = B.** Medications of persons needing assistance should be stored in a locked compartment away from other residents. Some residents wander and may be inclined to pick up belongings of others. The person needing assistance may accidentally, or for other reasons, lose the medications.

4. **Correct answer = D.** HIPAA states the facility must have a Notice of Privacy Practices that states how the facility protects the privacy, confidentiality, and security of residents' records.

5. **Correct answer = A.** The risk agreement is a document that provides for the resident to state the behavior that may be harmful but that the resident takes responsibility for and any consequences of the behavior. The agreement acknowledges the resident's right to refuse treatment.

6. **Correct answer = C.** The living will and power of attorney for healthcare are recognized documents used by persons to state their wishes regarding end-of-life care. A guardian or conservator is court appointed. The guardian has legal authority to act on behalf of, and make decisions for, the resident. The basic duty is to provide for the personal care and maintenance of the incapacitated person. A conservator is appointed to manage the estate of a protected person.

7. **Correct answer = D.** The behaviors of the resident are those usually exhibited by a person with depression. A precipitating cause is the resident's wife's death. Schizophrenia is a group of mental disorders requiring psychiatric treatment. Symptoms are very different from those exhibited by this resident. A person with a stroke has recognizable physical symptoms.

8. **Correct answer = B.** Mrs. Jones's symptoms are typical of a person experiencing delirium. It is not likely that Mrs. Jones is having a relapse after being treated. Recovery and hydration are positive states that should not cause a fever.

9. **Correct answer = C.** Residents and some theorists who have studied persons regarding activity claim that when people can continue activities the quality of their lives is maintained or improved. Activities in the community help residents to stay connected to their previous lifestyles. Activities in the facility help residents physically and psychosocially.

10. **Correct answer = C.** Your residents are your first concern, but you do not want to incent panic. Your disaster plan should have been discussed when the heavy rain had been going on for a week. No doubt your facility is in a flood area. Waiting for the water to arrive is courting disaster. The plan should include calm behavior of the department heads and staff and should identify the transportation company your facility will use. Calling the transportation company will confirm your need for evacuation. Your plan should also include your destination for residents and agreements for other items discussed in this chapter.

REFERENCES

Agency for Healthcare Research and Quality. National Institute of Mental Health. 2001. *Patient-Centered Care: Customizing Care to Meet Patients' Needs.* Washington, DC:

Agency for Healthcare Research and Quality.

Allen, J. 2004. *RC/AL Administration. The Knowledge Base.* 2nd ed. New York: Springer Publishing Company.

Alzheimer's Association. 2005. *Dementia Care Recommendations for RC/AL Residences and Nursing Homes.* Chicago: Alzheimer's Association.

American Association of Homes and Services for the Aging. Washington, DC.

American Association of Homes and Services for the Aging, American Senior Housing Association, Assisted Living Federation of America, National Center for Assisted Living, and National Investment Center for the Seniors Housing and Care Industry. 2006. *2006 Overview of Assisted Living.* Stratten Publishing & Marketing Inc.

American Society of Consultant Pharmacists. 2003. *Medication Management in Assisted Living. Assuring Accuracy of Medication Administration.* Alexandria, VA: American Society of Consultant Pharmacists.

Assisted Living Assessment Workgroup. 2003. *Assisted Living Workgroup Report to the US Senate Special Committee on Aging.* Washington, DC.

Assisted Living Federation of America. Publication Section. Alexandria, VA.

Center for Medicare Advocacy. 2003. *Center co-authors paper: Policy Principles for RC/AL (2005).* Washington, DC: Center for Medicare Advocacy.

Committee on Quality of Health Care in America. Institute for Health Care Improvement, Institute of Medicine. *Crossing the Quality Chasm: A New Health System for the 21st Century.* Washington, DC: National Academies Press.

Ebert, M., P. Larsen, B. Nucombe. 2000. *Diagnosis and Treatment in Psychiatry.* New York: Lange Medical Books/McGraw-Hill.

Erikson, E. 1963. *Childhood and Society.* 2nd ed. New York: W.W. Norton & Company.

Goldman, H. 2000. *Review of General Psychiatry.* 5th ed. New York: McGraw-Hill.

Linton, A., and H. Lach. 2006. *Mattheson & McConnell's Gerontological Nursing.* 3rd ed. New York: Elsevier.

Mollica, R. 2003. *Testimony before Senate Special Committee on Aging.*

National Center for Assisted Living. 2006. *Assisted Living State Regulatory Review.* Washington, DC: National Center for Assisted Living.

National Hospice and Palliative Care Organization. 2000. *A Handout.*

National Institutes of Health. 1998. *Consensus Development Program: Rehabilitation.* Washington, DC: National Institutes of Health.

Public Housing and Seniors Housing Service Models.

Slee's Health Care Terms, Third Comprehensive Edition.

Steffens, D., G. Blazer, and W. Busse. 2004. *The American Psychiatric Publishing Textbook of Geriatric Psychiatry.* Arlington, VA: American Psychiatric Publishing Company.

Thomas, W. 2004. *What are Old People for? How Elders will Change the World.* Acton, MA: VanderWyk & Burnham.

Thorson, J. 2000. *Aging in a Changing Society.* 2nd ed. New York: Brunner-Routledge.

U.S. Department of Agriculture. 2005. Steps to a healthier you. MyPyramid.com.

U.S. Department of Health and Human Services. 1999. *A National Study of Assisted Living.* Washington, DC: U.S. Department of Health and Human Services.

Waye, A. 2005. ALFs strengthen community bonds. *Provider* 32(7): 25–37.

Witmer, D. 2005. *Assistance with Medications.* Boise, ID: Idaho Health Care Association.

SUGGESTED READINGS

Eliopoulis, C. 2005. *Gerontological Nursing.* 6th ed. Philadelphia, PA: Lippincott, Williams, & Wilkins.

Gold, M. 2004. Designs for extended living. *Provider* 30(11): 18–33.

Taylor, H. 2005. *Assessing the Nursing and Care Needs of Older Adults: A Patient-Centered Approach.* Ashland, OH: Radcliffe Publishing.

Willging, P. 2004. I've Learned About Long-Term Care's Reality, Thanks to My Mom. *Provider* 53(11): 15–17.

Worland, K. (2006). *RC/AL Director. News, Best Practices & Professional Development for Assisted Living Administrators.* Bethesda, MD: Praxsys, Inc.

Zimmerman, S., Ann L. Gruber-Baldini, Philip D. Sloane, J. Kevin Eckert, J. Richard Hebel, Leslie A. Morgan, Sally C. Stearns, Judith Wildfire, Jay Magaziner, Cory Chen, and Thomas R. Konrad. 2003. Assisted Living and Nursing Homes: Apples and Oranges? *The Gerontologist* 43: 107–116. Special Issue.

IMPORTANT WEB SITES

- American Association of Homes and Services for the Aging. http://www.aahsa.org
- American College of Health Care Administrators. http://www.achca.org
- American Health Care Association and National Center for Assisted Living. http://www.ahca.org
- Assisted Living Federation of America. http://www.alfa.org
- Concise definitions/descriptions and information about numerous topics. http://en.wikipedia.org
- Description of RC/AL models of care. http://www.housingresearch.org
- Medicaid and Medicare. http://www.medicare.gov
- National Center for Assisted Living. http://www.ncal.org
- National Hospice and Palliative Care Organization. http://www.nho.org
- Patient-centered care overview. http://www.cmwf.org
- Person-Centered Care: Customizing Care to Meet Patients' Needs. http://grants.nih.gov
- Person-centered care for persons with disabilities. http://www.moddrc.com
- Rehabilitation of brain-injured persons (TBI). http://consensus.nih.gov/1998/1998TraumaticBrainInjury109html.htm
- Robert Mollica's Report to the Senate Committee On Aging. http://aging.senate.gov/public/-files/hr98rm.pdf
- U.S. Department of Agriculture food pyramid. http://www.mypyramid.org

ROBERT VAN DYK is president and CEO of Van Dyk Health Care, which owns and operates two nursing homes, two assisted living residences, senior housing with 62 congregate care apartments, a rehabilitation company, and a health and fitness center. He is a founder and principal of Assisted Living Training Associates (ALTA), a professional organization specializing in the training of assisted living administrators and ancillary personnel. Currently, Mr. Van Dyk is the secretary/treasurer of the American Health Care Association (AHCA) and the immediate past chairman of the National Center for Assisted Living (NCAL). He serves on the executive committee and board of governors of both associations.

CHAPTER 4

HUMAN RESOURCES MANAGEMENT

Robert Van Dyk

Introduction

Human resource management is the traditional title used to describe the effective and efficient management of the people we employ in residential care/assisted living (RC/AL) facilities, whether we're publicly traded or a small, independent residence. Most would agree that managing our organizations is becoming ever more difficult and the ability to recruit and retain good, loyal staff represents one of the greatest challenges our profession will face in the years ahead. I believe our success in attracting and keeping the best people will depend on the quality and effectiveness of the leadership we provide. As we enter the 21st century, we begin to think in terms of *human resource leadership*. Although most textbooks continue to use the term *human resource management*, in today's environment our goal is to lead our employees. We manage things; we lead people. The obvious question, then, is, what's the best way to lead people? The textbook answers of many managers might be the following:

- To recruit and retain staff
- To operate efficiently
- To make certain care is delivered

We must lead our staff to ensure quality resident care is provided in our assisted living residences. When I say *lead our staff*, I mean we must care for our employees. We must create a happy and loyal staff. If our staff is happy, our residents and their families will be happy. If they are happy, you will have a successful RC/AL facility.

The leadership of your staff may be delegated to other individual(s). However, the responsibility for establishing the environment in which these people work is yours. The way your leadership team leads their staff is up to you. You must develop your own method of monitoring their performance. The way you lead your employees will and should be reflected in the way they treat and lead their direct staff, and that attitude will be reflected in the quality of care that is delivered. The best place to start is with the example you set. You cannot lead your management team one way and expect them to lead their staff differently. You must be their role model.

Job Description

Prior to recruiting for an open or newly created position, or interviewing prospective candidates, or hiring a new employee, you should have a **job description** for the position to be filled. This document should give an overall view of the responsibilities of the job, as well as the skills needed to perform the job successfully.

The job description should include at least the following:

- Title of position.
- Department under which the position works.
- Supervisor or title of individual to whom the position reports.
- Salary or wage (exempt or nonexempt).
- Pay grade (hourly or annually). Some employers present the salary as weekly

37

or monthly so that interviewees do not attempt to interpret the annual salary as an implied contract for one year.

- Job summary—keep it short.
- Essential/primary job responsibilities. This should be a very specific list or description of the primary functions the employee is expected to complete.
- Secondary responsibilities. This section includes those functions the employee may be asked to assist or participate in outside the immediate scope of the primary job.
- Skills and qualifications. This should be a list of any educational degrees, licenses, certifications, or special training required of a successful applicant. Other skills such as verbal or written proficiency, computer skills, or other technical or managerial skills necessary to performing this position are also listed here.
- Experience. This portion of the document lists years of experience required or requested of the applicant.
- Supervisory duties. The approximate number of employees and their respective job titles are found here.
- Equipment to be used.
- Physical requirements to do the job. This section is important because of the **Americans with Disabilities Act (ADA)**. As an employer, your requirement to make reasonable accommodations for employees with a disability may rest with the minimum physical requirements of the position as stated in your job description.
- Work conditions. If there are any unusual, dangerous, or stressful working conditions expected in this job position and of the applicant, they should be noted here. For example: Position requires applicant to clean windows, gutters, chimneys, and roofs using a 30-foot ladder. Similarly, if there is hazardous waste or strong chemicals that must be handled, this too should be articulated in this section of the job description.

Staff Recruitment

Newspaper advertisements are the most commonly used means of soliciting and making people aware of job openings. However, a valuable but often overlooked source of new employees is word of mouth. If you have created an environment that has produced a happy and loyal staff, these people can be your best source of finding other employees with similar attitudes and values. In my experience, I have found that employees recommend co-workers who are also willing to carry their share of the workload. Employees also tend to monitor those they have recommended because providing a recommendation for someone who does not perform well can be seen as a poor reflection on the original employee.

If you are opening a new property and need to recruit a large workforce, the job fair is an excellent vehicle. Held at your property or at a local restaurant, it can be a very effective way to bring in large numbers of people over one or two days. Serve light refreshments and set up stations for each department where members of your leadership team can meet the prospects and explain the position and your expectations.

The Internet is growing in popularity as a cost-effective way of filling positions. There are Web sites where care aides can look for jobs, companies offer certified nursing assistant (CNA) training, and other opportunities are available. When people move from one state another, the Web is good place to look for jobs and let potential employers know they are coming into the area and want to work with elderly persons.

How will we find good people? Terms some human resource professionals are now using are *value propositions* and *branding*. What they are asking is how we can create a corporate culture that is unique and that sets us apart from our competitors? Companies must become creative in establishing schedules for staff. You should try to find part-time staff whose personal schedules fit the needs of your assisted living residents. Examples include stay-at-home moms/dads who are available while the children are in school, college students who have classes only three days a week, or school teachers who can work summers and holidays.

Millennials

As we face the challenges of recruitment and retention, we would be well advised to better understand who members of the future workforce will be and how we can best attract and retain them. As noted earlier, the Baby Boomers are on their way out and the Gen Xers are here but represent the smallest population group. The next large group we must prepare for are the Millennials. This generational group was born between 1980 and 2000 and is nearly as large as the Baby Boom generation. One author describes the Millennials as "sociable, optimistic, talented, well-educated, collaborative, open-minded, influential, and achievement oriented." (Raines 2003.) As a group, they have been raised to believe they are "sought after, needed, and indispensable." As they enter the workforce, they are expected to come with higher expectations than the generations before them had. Millennials, also known as the "Internet Generation," tend to let many people know of their displeasure or how impressed they are with a company through the many forms of electronic communication available to them. (Raines 2003.)

Millennials are unlike recent generations. Many believe they will make the most significant contributions to society in our history. Claire Raines, an expert in sociological demographics, believes the following six principles will be key to managing the Millennials:

1. **You be the leader.** This generation has grown up with structure and supervision, with parents who were role models. The Millennials are looking for leaders with honesty and integrity. It's not that they don't want to be leaders themselves; they'd just like some great role models first.

2. **Challenge me.** Millennials want learning opportunities. They want to be assigned to projects they can learn from. They're looking for growth, development, a career path.

3. **Let me work with friends.** Millennials say they want to work with people they *click* with. They like being friends with coworkers. Employers who provide for the social aspects of work will find those efforts well rewarded by this newest cohort. Some companies are even interviewing and hiring groups of friends.

4. **Let's have fun.** A little humor, a bit of silliness, even a little irreverence will make your work environment more attractive.

5. **Respect me.** "Treat our ideas respectfully," they ask, "even though we haven't been around a long time."

6. **Be flexible.** The busiest generation ever isn't going to give up its activities just because of jobs. A rigid schedule is a sure-fire way to lose your Millennial employees. (Raines 2003)

Universal Worker

The universal worker (UW) is a position many assisted living residences have found to be effective. Generally, the UW is a resident care aide whose duties and responsibilities go beyond meeting only the personal care needs of the resident. The UW is involved in the housekeeping of a resident's room, participates in the activities offered, as well as serves and cleans up the dining room. Depending on the home, this position may include more or fewer responsibilities.

The UW position can be the most effective way to offer quality and continuity. The UW has the opportunity to know the resident in all settings and make observations relative to each. Helping residents get up in the morning and assisting with their activities of daily living

(ADLs—bathing, grooming, dressing, toileting, etc.) enables the UW to observe any physical needs and/or changes in residents that occur. Cleaning residents' rooms gives the UW a glimpse into another part of the residents' world, which can be instructive in understanding them.

The concept of universal worker may not be right for everyone. Some states may have regulations that will not allow for this type of position. The final decision on how you staff your facility should always be based on how you can best meet the needs of your residents. In the end, that is what it's all about.

Immigration and 9/11

The terrorist attacks on September 11, 2001, affected our nation in innumerable ways. We as employers have always had the responsibility to hire only legal aliens. Since 9/11, the pressure on employers to do so has increased. It is illegal to knowingly hire any individual who is not eligible to work in the United States. If a potential employee lies and forges the required documentation, you may not be held liable. But taking the position of "don't ask, don't tell" is not an acceptable defense.

Employers must check and verify all documents to determine if a person is permitted to work in the United States. Proof of work eligibility is required of all employees and is accomplished by completing Form I-9. As an employer, you can request I-9 forms from the U.S. Citizenship and Immigration Service, which is part of the Department of Homeland Security. Employees must complete an I-9 form within three days of being hired.

Staffing Levels

There is no formula for staffing an assisted living residence. Every state has different requirements for staff qualifications, numbers of staff, and levels of care permitted to be delivered.

A general guideline to follow when determining your staffing is this: provide sufficient staff with the appropriate licensure, certification, and training to meet the needs of your residents based on the **acuity** of care residents require.

Interviewing

The first rule in interviewing a prospective employee is: do not ask yes and no questions. Also, avoid talking about yourself. This is your opportunity to learn about the applicant. Ask questions that give you an insight into the person. Some questions to ask might include the following:

1. Tell me a little about yourself.
2. Why are you leaving your present job?
3. Why are you interested in this job?
4. Why are you interested in this company?
5. Why do you believe you're qualified for this position?
6. Regarding your last job, what did you like best and least about it?
7. What was the most difficult problem you faced at your last job, and how did you handle it?
8. What are your greatest weaknesses?
9. What do you want to be doing five years from now?
10. What are your assets/best talents?
11. Why should we hire you for this position?
12. What qualities do you appreciate in a supervisor?
13. What did you think of your last employer?
14. What did you think of your last supervisor?
15. Why do you want to work with elderly people?
16. Do you have any questions?

Other questions you might consider are these:

- Education. Tell me about your degree(s). What was your favorite course? Tell me about your major and why you picked it.
- Personality traits
  - Describe yourself.
  - How would your previous employer or supervisor describe you?
  - What types of people upset you?
- Lifestyle. How do you spend your leisure time?
- Prior job questions
  - How did you get your previous job?
  - What were your responsibilities and duties?
  - Tell me about your supervisor.
  - Tell me about your major disappointment with that job.

The interview can be the best place to identify the right person for an open position. This is also an area where you can get into trouble. Affirmative Action and the Equal Employment Opportunity Commission (EEOC) have guidelines that prohibit employers from asking certain questions. Generally, you cannot ask questions regarding the following topics:

- National origin
- Religion, name of church, minister, priest, rabbi, etc.
- Religious holidays applicant observes
- Marital status or information about children
- A woman's maiden name
- Plans to start a family
- Sexual preference
- Financial or banking issues
- If an applicant rents or owns his/her residence
- Service in the military
- Previous arrests
- Age and date of birth
- Birthplace
- If the person has ever been treated for specific conditions. If the person has any disabilities.

The interview is a critical step in hiring your employees and proper functioning of your facility. Take the time to find the right people. When you conduct the interview, be prepared and respect the time the applicant has taken to meet with you. Consider what you would do or say if someone walks in seeking employment and doesn't have an appointment. What would you do or say if someone looking for a room for his or her mother walked in without an appointment? Each individual is valuable to the future of your home. Treat each with the same respect. You need to identify and hire the best people to care for the residents who have been entrusted to you. Never miss an opportunity to make them part of your team.

Retention

Assisted living residences retain their employees by maintaining low turnover rates. Employees generally stay with one employer for one or more of the following reasons:

- No other jobs are available in the marketplace.
- Compensation and benefit package are the best in the marketplace.
- Staff enjoy working at that home.

The first two reasons are somewhat obvious. The third, however, goes beyond good wages alone. The question I'd like to explore is, why does staff enjoy working at one home over another? Please consider the following philosophical and operational commitments on the part of management. Management:

1. Makes certain the first impression of their home is positive. Greet and treat prospective employees as the valued asset they are, from the time they walk in to apply for a job throughout the time they are employed.
2. Understands the needs and expectations of job applicants. Make certain potential employees know what your expectations are as well.

41

3. Creates a physical environment in which the staff enjoys working. Seriously consider developing a first-class employee lounge and/or break room. You may install air conditioning and a TV and DVD player/VCR in the staff lounge, or install air conditioning in the laundry and the kitchen where temperatures can get quite hot and uncomfortable.
4. Wants staff to feel valued, respected, appreciated, and empowered.
5. Recognizes employees for outstanding performance.
6. Compensates employees fairly. You don't need to pay the highest rate to create a loyal staff, but you must be competitive and fair.
7. Encourages and supports camaraderie among staff.
8. Makes the workplace fun.
9. Communicates clearly and often with staff on all shifts.
10. Offers opportunities for advancement (this topic is addressed in more detail later in this chapter).

Because of the increasing mobility of today's workforce, some companies create staying bonuses and incentive plans that require staff to remain with the company a certain amount of time to collect the bonus. In more extreme cases, some companies have offered auto and homeowners insurance or have even prepaid legal services. In the larger business world, some companies have created a new position called a "retention manager" to oversee programs for increasing employee retention. If you, as the owner or director of an assisted living facility, embrace the suggestions discussed in this chapter but your management/leadership staff does not, employee turnover will continue to be a challenge at your facility. Your leadership team must know how to lead and communicate with your staff, or turnover issues will not improve.

Opportunities for advancement are a very effective way to promote staff retention.

Many positions available in assisted living homes do not require employees to have special licensure or advanced degrees, and these positions have starting wages close to the minimum required by law. To the extent possible, work at creating ladders within each department and each position to give staff the opportunity to learn new skills and earn more money. One example is the "clinical laddering structure" where a resident care aide can go "up the ladder" and become a trainer or mentor for new aides. This aide could also become a lead care aide that supervises and schedules other aides. Depending on regulations in your state, the aide could continue up the ladder and go on to become a certified medication aide who is permitted to administer medications. Some aides have continued on to nursing school to become licensed practical nurses or registered nurses. Opportunities for advancement can be found in all departments; this is just one example. The significance of creating opportunities for advancement is that people don't feel they are trapped in a dead-end job and begin to lose interest. Boredom causes people to start looking for something new, and sometimes it manifests as poor attendance, poor attitude, or poor quality care.

Staff Recognition

People want to be recognized and praised for their work. You can praise people in many ways and only some are monetary—not all praise has to cost you money. Four ways to praise people at no cost are to offer personal praise, public praise, written praise, and electronic praise. In a study conducted by Bob Nelson (1994), these four types of recognition ranked in the top 10 ways people like to be praised.

Recognition is one of the most highly sought after wants and needs of your staff. It can also be one of the least expensive employee benefit you offer. You and your leadership team must make a conscious and concerted effort to recognize and reward your staff continually.

Compensation and Benefits

Compensation

When establishing a compensation and benefit package, it is critical to make certain all employees are treated equally. Obviously, that does not mean they all receive the same compensation. It does mean, however, that like positions receive similar wages that reflect experience, years of service, and other circumstances such as shift, holidays, and weekends worked, and so forth.

An employer can establish wages in different ways. The Bureau of Labor Statistics (a division of the U.S. Department of Labor) produces salary surveys. Trade associations and consultants also publish wage and salary surveys for their members and clients. Generally, these types of documents have limited applications. National surveys can act as a guide or give you reference salary ranges, but they are rarely germane to the specific marketplace in which you operate.

Another respected source of compensation information is the Hay system for evaluating jobs. The Hay methodology measures each job classification and its "relative weight" in the company. The system involves a complicated scoring matrix and requires knowledgeable management and human resource people to use it, factors that tend to restrict its use to larger corporations. The use of a numeric ranking system also creates a hierarchy by establishing one position as a rank or grade 1 position, while another position is a 2, 5, or 18. Some believe such ranking is not conducive to the team approach where everyone is considered an equally valuable member of the resident care team. However, the Hay system evaluates the job position as opposed to the individual doing the job. In the end, it generates a ranking of positions and pay grade ranges for employers to use when considering a new employee's wage or salary.

Some believe the Hay system is the "most widely used in the world," but the size, ownership, and operating model of your home will dictate which type of system is best suited for you.

Another approach widely used by smaller assisted living providers is to do a local market survey by job position. This can be accomplished with the cooperation of your peers that operate in your market area. Whether you are establishing a wage and benefit schedule for the first time or updating your current one, you must know what the competition is offering so that you can remain competitive in your marketplace. Some general factors to consider when you set pay scales include the following:

- Licensure required for the position
- Skills or experience you believe is necessary
- Availability of the type of person you are trying to hire or position you are trying to fill
- What you currently pay similar positions in your company
- Special conditions such as shifts, travel, and so forth
- Fringe benefits that your company offers, especially those benefits not customarily offered in assisted living facilities or in your marketplace

Benefits

The significance and value of your benefits should not be overlooked. Some of the more common benefits offered today include the following:

- Paid holiday time off
- Paid vacation
- Health insurance; most companies pay for a portion, and a few still pay 100 percent
- Paid jury duty
- Paid sick time
- Life insurance
- Retirement programs such as a 401(k)

Less common but also offered include the following:

- Educational assistance
- Long term disability
- Dental care
- Paid personal leave
- Paid maternity leave

Salary versus Hourly (Exempt vs. Nonexempt)

The Fair Labor Standards Act (FLSA) defines specific guidelines that help specify which employees are *exempt* from overtime and which are *nonexempt*. The FLSA requires employers to pay nonexempt employees overtime at the rate of one and one-half times their hourly wage, if they have worked more than 40 hours in a week. However, the FLSA doesn't require overtime for working more than 8 hours in a day. Some states have additional rules governing overtime that you should review prior to establishing your own policy.

Equal Pay for Equal Work

Under both the FLSA and the Equal Pay Act of 1963, employers must pay men and women equally if they are both doing the same job. Job titles have not been found to be the deciding factor. The courts, in deciding equal jobs, have looked at the work duties, skill levels required, and working conditions. The Equal Pay Act does permit wage and benefit differences based on the following factors:

- Years of service
- Performance
- Pay tied to production quantity or quality
- Experience level

Contract versus At-Will Employees

Elsewhere in this chapter, I discuss **employment-at-will**. Most states recognize this concept, which specifies people who work at the will of the company. They have no contract that guarantees or binds them to the company. In other words, either party, the employer or the employee, can terminate the relationship at any time and for any reason. You can fire at-will employees, or they can quit without cause.

The opposite of at-will employment is employees who have an employment contract, which is a legally enforceable document. In the contract, the employee and employer agree to a fixed amount of time the working relationship will exist. The contract can be severed only for cause or predetermined conditions. An example of this is a marketing department employee whose contract specifies a certain census must be maintained or a specific number of leads must be generated within a certain period of time; if the contract conditions are not met, the employer can terminate the contract.

If you must make a financial investment in the development or training of a new employee, you may want to create a contract with the employee to protect that investment. For example, if the employee leaves before a specified time, you can recoup the investment.

The letter you write to welcome a new employee should be carefully written so as not to imply some commitment for a long tenure. For example, avoid including such sentence as this: "We look forward to you joining our organization and know we will enjoy many years working together." In the courtroom, it could be argued that the preceding sentence implies the employee was offered a long term position.

It has become necessary for employers to thoroughly understand anything to do with employees and the hiring process, and all policies and procedures as well as documents should be reviewed by legal counsel. The training of each member of your leadership team must include information on **human resources** issues and labor laws. Members of your leadership team are the men and women who will be closest to your staff. Their knowledge of these issues can be your best defense of your greatest liability.

Unions

To date, only a small number of assisted living residences have been unionized successfully, perhaps because assisted living is the "new kid" in the long term care continuum. Or perhaps it is because of size. Generally, the more employees a company has, the greater the risk of poor communication and unionization.

Regarding unions, you should always consult a labor attorney to guide you in how to prevent unionization, how to deal with a union organizing drive, and how to conduct union contract negotiations. Some very clear guidelines must be followed when dealing with unions. Failure to do so can create significant problems and loss of rights in the process.

Staff Orientation and Staff Training

Too often, implementing a thorough orientation, employee training, and ongoing retraining program is viewed as expensive with a concern that it will not yield substantial dividends. Nothing could be further from the truth. Some owners fear they will spend a substantial sum of money on a new employee, and then the new hire will leave before the organization can recoup the expense. Perhaps this might happen, but the only thing worse is to hire staff who are ill prepared, perform poorly, and stay.

The first step in training begins with orientation. This is an opportunity to review many of the basic policies and procedures in place, the company mission and vision, the organizational structure, and the requirements of the job. Avoid jamming too much information into a short time period.

Make certain the individual or department heads who provide orientation embody the culture and spirit of your company/home. Those leading and teaching should act as role models and display the type of enthusiasm, commitment, loyalty, and work ethic you would like to see all of your staff display.

The first task in new employee orientation is to create a fun nonthreatening environment. Many people are nervous when they start a new job. Consider some warm-up exercises or games to get the class laughing and feeling more at ease. Then, review the history of the company they have decided to join. People like to know who started the company and why. Answer such questions as if the company has other locations and if it has plans for opening more homes, and where. Knowing the company's past and plans for the future can give new employees a sense of pride and ownership, as well as a feeling that opportunities to move up or around the company exist. An effective way to demonstrate opportunities for growth and upward mobility in the company is to introduce new employees to members of your leadership team who started at the company with entry-level jobs and worked their way up to managerial positions (this is an example of the job ladder concept discussed earlier in the chapter). The opportunities for advancement can encourage lower turnover and more long term employees.

Next, review the organizational chart. The type you use is a personal choice. The traditional hierarchical type with the president on top and showing boxes and lines going down the chart is accurate and effective. On the other hand, it also has a tendency to imply the positions toward the top of the chart are more important than the positions closer to the bottom.

Another diagrammatic representation of the organization is a circle with the customer/ resident/family at the core. This chart looks like a wheel with spokes. This approach reinforces the fact that the resident is the center of the organization's attention and the focus. It shows that everyone contributes, each in their own unique way, to patient-centered care.

45

The way you choose to explain where and how each employee fits into the organization is your choice, but it is one of the areas you should cover early in the orientation process.

Work Environment and Expectations

New staff have many questions about their new job. Often, the questions are more basic than you might imagine. Don't overlook the obvious issues. Start with a tour of the building(s) staff in which new staff will work—no one wants to get lost the first day on the job. If possible, conduct different portions of the orientation in different parts of the building. Tour the building each day of orientation.

Tours should always include where employees are to enter and exit the building, where they punch in and out on a time clock, where the employee lounge or break room is, which restrooms staff are permitted to use, and the location of their respective departments. This information should all be included early on and throughout orientation.

A successful orientation program uses a variety of teaching tools. Class feedback and involvement should be encouraged. Allow adequate time to cover all the material. Do not rush. The human mind can absorb only so much information. Yes, there is a cost to the company for each day or extra day spent on orientation or training. I suggest you look at this as an investment in resident care, not as an expense to the company.

Employee Handbook/Personnel Policies

The employee handbook can be an excellent and effective tool for communicating the rules, guidelines, and culture of your company. However, it must be unique to your organization. You need to articulate those factors that are important to the way in which your organization operates.

An employee handbook does the following:

- Encourages the consistent treatment of all staff regardless of job title

- Is a convenient reference tool for prospective and existing employees
- Is useful in developing a better understanding of the corporate culture
- Is a simple summary of your expectations of staff performance and behavior
- Is an effective way to ensure you are in compliance with notification rules relative to most, if not all, employee/employer labor laws, such as sexual harassment, equal employment, family leave, and so forth

After employees have received the employee handbook, you must require them to sign an acknowledgment that they have read, understand, and agree to perform their job in accordance with the handbook.

In recent years, employee handbooks have been used against employers, and courts have upheld claims that the handbook was an employment contract that limits the employer's right to terminate an employee. Experts have recommended the following procedures to mitigate the risk of your manual being construed as a contract:

- Include prominent disclaimers that the handbook is not a contract and is not intended to alter the at-will status of any employee.
- Make it clear the handbook is meant only to be a source of information and is subject to change at any time without prior notification.
- Let employees know they may resign at any time and the organization may discharge an employee at any time, with or without cause.
- Include a statement that the company is not compelled to follow the disciplinary procedures outlined in the handbook and that the company might not consistently apply all disciplinary procedures.
- Avoid words, promises, or guarantees that imply the company will take specific action in certain circumstances.

Table 4.1 is a checklist of those items to be included in your employee handbook. This table is meant only as a guide; each home should make certain its handbook reflects the personality, policies, and culture of the ownership. One size does not fit all.

Personnel Files/Records

There are many reasons to maintain personnel records, not the least of which is that some employment documents, such as Form I-9 and wage and hour records, must be maintained for specific time periods as required by law. It is important, although not required, to retain numerous other documents to prove evidence of legal compliance or to create a history of an employee's performance, job description, disciplinary actions, promotions, and so forth. These records should be stored and maintained in one secure area, and the filing cabinets should be locked at all times. It is wise to decide in advance which records are important and create a checklist to ensure you have what you need. If you're not careful, the filing can become very large, unwieldy, and difficult to manage.

The most common files you might maintain include the following:

- Employment application, along with supporting materials such as resume, transcripts, and interview notes
- Recommendation letters and reference checks
- Copies of restrictive covenants with employee's prior employers

Table 4.1 Employee Handbook Checklist		
The Company • Corporate philosophy • Job descriptions • Mission statement • Organizational chart **Issues of Pay and Performance** • Attendance policies • Changes in employee status • Employee classifications • Exit reviews • Hiring policies • Hiring of relatives • Hours of operation • Issues of pay • Outside employment • Performance review • Reduction in staff • References • Reimbursement for expenses • Salary reviews • Termination • Use of personal vehicles • Work hours	**Benefits** • Appointments • Dental insurance • Disability income • Doctor and dental • Employment assistance program • Employment education • Extended benefits after leaving the company (e.g., pensions) • Family and medical leave • Funeral leave • General leaves of absence • Health insurance • Holidays • Jury duty • Life insurance • Military leave • Personal leave • Sharing of company profits • Sick leave • Training • Unemployment compensation • Vacation • Workers' compensation	**Standards of Conduct** • Disciplinary appeals • Disciplinary procedures • Grievance procedures • Involuntary termination • Problem resolution • Process • Voluntary termination **General Information** • Alcohol on company premises or on business travel • Business gifts • Company property • Company vehicles • Confidential nature of business • Contributions for gifts • Emergency and safety procedures • Other contributions • Personal mail/e-mail • Personal property • Personnel records • Sexual harassment • Smoking/chewing tobacco • Telephone procedures • Traffic and parking violations • Vehicle liability coverage

- Offer letter and any contractual documents, such as restrictive covenants, arbitration agreements, and so on
- Form I-9
- Copy of New Hire Report form
- Tax withholding forms (W-4, W-5, and state equivalents)
- Job description, including statement as to whether position is exempt or nonexempt
- Copies of any required licenses or certificates required for the position
- Documentation of receipt of employee handbook
- Testing materials, if the employee was required to take any tests as part of the application process
- Training records relating to job competency, safety, sexual harassment policies, and so forth
- Evaluations
- Commendations and disciplinary actions
- Pay records
- Personal information—home address, home telephone number, name of spouse, and emergency contact
- Benefit plan participation records (application, beneficiary designation, etc.)
- Exit interview notes
- Recommendation letters and notes of references given to prospective employers

Some experts suggest you keep in the personnel file only information that legally can be used as the basis for an employment-related decision. Employment decisions include hiring, firing, promotion, demotion, layoff, training opportunities, and all other actions taken regarding employees. Employment decisions may *not* be made on the basis of sex, race, national origin, color, religion, or veteran's status, so keep all **equal employment opportunity** records separate. Making decisions based on a person's disability status also is illegal, so keep all medical information separate (there are privacy issues here as well). Garnishment orders cannot be used as a basis

for employment decisions, so all paperwork having to do with garnishment must be kept separate. I-9 forms must be made available on demand to Department of Labor inspectors, and it is best to keep them in a separate place for convenience.

Record Retention

Not all records carry the same requirement for retention. Table 4.2 provides a succinct guide to the most common records and their respective retention periods.

Access to Employee Files

Employee Access

Some states have laws that ensure employees have the right to see their personnel files as well as copy and contest any negative evaluations or comments recorded. For example, the state of California has an interesting approach. California state law allows employees to view their files, but employees can make copies only of those documents the employee signed. This is one way to ensure all evaluations and disciplinary actions are signed!

Allowing access is generally thought to be advisable. Without access, an air of distrust can be created. Allowing access enhances open communication and a more productive, less secretive relationship between the administrator and staff. Most important, open access makes your managers more conscious of what they write and more diligent in maintaining thorough records on each employee.

Outside Access

The personnel record belongs to the company. The information in it is confidential and should not be divulged to anyone outside the company, such as a bank requesting income verification for a loan, without the express written consent of the employee. Within the

Table 4.2 Records to Keep and the Recommended Number of Years to Keep Them		
Record	**Years**	**Notes**
Hiring Records* Job applications, resumes Records relating to refusal to hire Advertisements about openings, promotions, or training opportunities *Federal contractors should keep these records for at least 2 years.	1 year	Keep equal employment opportunity (EEO) information separate
Basic Employee Information I-9 for all Work permits for minors	3 years after hire or 1 year after termination, whichever is later	Keep I-9s separate
Payroll Records Name, address, SSN Date of birth Job classification Amounts and dates of payments Daily and weekly hours Overtime hours and pay Annuity and pension payments Benefits, deductions and additions	4 years	
Tax Records	4 years	
Employment Actions Hires, separations, rehires Promotions, demotions Transfers, layoffs, recalls Training opportunities Employment test results	1 year from date of action	
Health, Medical, Safety Data Job-related illnesses and injuries Requests for accommodation of disability Medical exams Toxic substance exposure records Blood-borne pathogen exposure records Family Medical Leave Act (FMLA)	5 years 1 year 30 years 30 years 30 years 3 years	

company, it is advisable to restrict access to an as-needed basis.

Employee Evaluations

Generally, companies evaluate new hires within 90 days of hiring. It is generally accepted that the first 90 days is a probationary period, and it is far easier to discharge an employee without cause during that time.

Check your state laws on this issue. For the first 30 days, employees should be observed closely, for the next 30 days they should be monitored and provided more training, and then in the last 30 days permanent employment should be decided on with their three-month evaluation.

The annual evaluation serves a number of purposes. The most obvious is to review the employee's performance and determine the size or amount of a pay increase. It is also an opportunity to discuss how well an employee has performed and those areas in which the employee must improve. If an employee's performance has not been satisfactory, the annual evaluation should not be the first time the employee hears about it. The annual evaluation is the time to recap and discuss how please or displease you are with the person's progress.

I call a simple but effective outline for a performance evaluation the Four As—ability, attendance, attitude, and appearance:

- **Ability.** In this portion of the evaluation, you discuss the employee's performance. In this section, discuss the person's abilities, your expectations of the employee, and the employee's expectations of you as an employer.
- **Attendance.** In some homes, employee attendance can become a chronic problem if not addressed. Most homes have their own unique way of dealing with it. The bottom line is, if staff do not arrive at work on time, they are short changing you, increasing the workload of their fellow employees, and most important, not giving high-quality care to the residents who are paying the bills.

  Poor attendance can be an indicator of many things, including poor organizational skills, staying out too late the night before, personal or family problems, working another job and not being able to get to your home on time, or lack of interest or commitment to the job. Address these issues as appropriate in this section of the evaluation.
- **Attitude.** The attitudes staff display to others significantly affects the satisfaction of your residents. For example, would you like to be greeted each day with a happy and warm smile, a cheery and uplifting voice, and a positive attitude toward life, or would you be satisfied being cared for by someone who acts as though he or she doesn't want to

be at work, he or she is doing you a favor, and who sees the glass as half empty?

Frederick Reichheld (1996), in his book *The Loyalty Effect*, found through his study of corporate loyalty, that 68 percent of customers leave or do not return because of an attitude of indifference exhibited by company employees.

Employees with positive attitudes create a more positive and happy work environment. Happy employees are more loyal, and more loyal staff stay with you longer, which equates to low turnover. Because staff attitude is so important to every aspect of your operation, address it in the annual performance review.

- **Appearance.** An assisted living facility has only one chance to make a first impression. This relates to the appearance of your staff as well as their attitude.

  Some assisted living residences have dress codes, some supply uniforms, and others have dress guidelines. No matter what your policy is on dress and appearance, it is important to understand you need to have a policy and to enforce it. Address an employee's appearance in this section of the evaluation.

The Four As are general guidelines for creating important pieces of the **performance appraisal**. You may choose different words or categories of performance to evaluate, but realize the employee evaluation is an important tool that, when used properly, only enhances the quality of care provided in your homes. Experts in the field of human resources offer the following reasons to do a performance appraisal on all staff:

- Providing feedback to employees about their performance
- Determining who gets promoted
- Facilitating layoff or downsizing decisions
- Encouraging performance improvement
- Motivating superior performance
- Setting and measuring goals
- Counseling poor performers

- Determining compensation changes
- Encouraging coaching and mentoring
- Supporting human resource planning or succession planning
- Determining individual training and development needs
- Determining organizational training and development needs
- Confirming that good hiring decisions are being made
- Providing legal defensibility for personnel decisions
- Improving overall organizational performance

You can conduct employee appraisals in many different ways and forms. Although no laws require you evaluate employee performance, it is highly advisable that you do.

Discipline and Termination

Discipline

Most employee handbooks include a list of items that are cause for immediate dismissal. Some examples include the following:

- Resident abuse
- Theft
- Unauthorized use of property
- Striking a fellow employee
- Possession or use of illegal substances
- Possession or use of weapons
- Illegal gambling
- Violence or threats of violence against supervisors
- Use of company facilities to transmit obscene material
- Racial or sexual harassment
- Intentional discrimination
- Falsifying records or reports
- Willful disregard of important company policies

Other offenses may call for a multistep approach to discipline. The progressive process may include these steps:

Step 1. Oral warning in private
Step 2. Written warning
Step 3. Suspension without pay
Step 4. Demotion
Step 5. Termination

Examples of offenses appropriate for this process may include the following:

- Tardiness
- Excessive absenteeism
- Minor neglect at work
- Violation of company parking regulations
- Violation of smoking policies
- Violation of use of cell phones or personal calls on company time or equipment

Termination

You must make it clear to employees the reasons why disciplinary action will be initiated and under what circumstances discipline will be initiated. Beware that if your personnel policy states that an employee's job or position will "only be terminated for cause" (a very popular phrase used in most handbooks), you have just lost your at-will relationship and converted your handbook into an employment contract. With such wording, you can only terminate an employee for cause, and this is significant if you operate in a state that recognizes at-will employment, and most states do. Likewise, if your policy outlines a multistep disciplinary process and indicates these steps will be followed before more severe discipline is initiated, you must follow the steps exactly. If you don't, you can be sued and you will, in most cases, lose.

Terminating an employee is not a simple matter. This is good to the extent it protects employees from unethical or unfair employers and labor practices. Yet it has also created more and more lawsuits.

The most effective and generally safest approach to employee termination is to write up the language you plan to use in the event of a reference check, and have the employee sign and authorize its use. This generally releases the employer from liability and future claims of defamation.

The obvious area of cause for defamation is where the old employer calls the new employer and provides unsolicited, malicious, false, or intentionally damaging information that can be considered both retaliatory and defaming, and that would be cause for legal action.

Turnover

Recruiting and retaining staff usually is an ongoing process. Staff turnover is impossible to avoid. In your less skilled positions, annual turnover can be as much as 100 percent or more, and the turnover of executive directors is frighteningly high as well.

Turnover can be controlled by hiring the right person for the right job. An individual's personality and work ethic are more important than the skills he or she brings to the position. You can teach new skills and change existing skills, but it is nearly impossible to change attitude.

An important leadership tool is your "turnover report." As mentioned earlier, turnover is very expensive for an organization and in time has a deleterious effect on continuity, staff morale, and the quality of care you deliver. For these reasons, you should regularly monitor your staff turnover. Watch for trends by job title, shift, department, and most of all, team leader. As noted elsewhere in this chapter, no matter how much you pay, no one wants to work for a bad boss.

Whenever an employee leaves voluntarily, conduct an exit interview. Presumably, the outgoing employee will feel free to tell you exactly why he or she is leaving. This is an excellent opportunity for you to gain insight into why you are losing staff. Following are some questions to ask in the exit interview:

- Why have you decided to leave?
- Did you enjoy working at our home?
- Did you feel valued, respected, appreciated?

- Did you feel you were always treated fairly by your team leader?
- If you had problems or questions, was the appropriate member of the leadership team available and did that person meet your needs?
- Did you find the other staff you worked with pleasant and easy to get along with?
- Did you feel the orientation and subsequent training you received prepared you for your job?
- If you could make any changes in the way we operate, what would they be?

If your turnover is a result of a high number of people being fired, you need to explore this as well. If many people are fired, it could mean the selection process is flawed, the person responsible for selecting new staff doesn't have the necessary training and skills for that responsibility, or staff are not being trained adequately for their jobs and are unable to meet your expectations.

Regulations Guiding Human Resources Practices

Sarbanes-Oxley Act

In 2002, Congress passed the Sarbanes-Oxley Act. This legislation is targeted at and in response to the rash of corporate scandals in publicly traded companies such as Enron. Although the legislation is directed at publicly traded companies, most large organizations have chosen to adopt the intent if not actual portions of the law. The most widely adopted section has been the development of a corporate code of ethics. Some examples of issues covered by a company code of ethics are given in Table 4.3.

Another provision of Sarbanes-Oxley is the protection afforded to whistle-blowing. It is now a criminal offense for an employer to terminate or retaliate in any form against an employee who discloses the illegal practices of his or her employer. The whistle-blower's job is also protected if the person cooperates,

---

Table 4.3 Codes of Ethics

- Even if your company is not publicly traded and subject to the Sarbanes-Oxley Act, it is a good idea to have a company code of ethics that applies to all employees. In the code of ethics, you might address the following activities, many of which are illegal as well as unethical:

- Hiring relatives
- Carrying phantom employees
- Borrowing money from subordinate employees, vendors, or customers
- Accepting bribes, kickbacks, expensive gifts, or lavish entertainment from vendors or customers
- Accepting discounts on purchases from vendors or customers that are not offered to the general public
- Falsifying business records, tax returns, or reports to government agencies
- Carrying off-the-books accounts or funds
- Performing paid services for customers on a personal basis outside normal company channels
- Blacklisting employees, customers, or vendors
- Fixing bids or sharing pricing or cost information with competitors
- Requiring customers to buy unwanted products to get products they do want

---

testifies, or otherwise assists law enforcement investigations or Congress in the investigation of their employer.

Civil Rights Act—Title VII

Title VII is a provision of the Civil Rights Act of 1964 that prohibits discrimination in virtually every employment circumstance on the basis of race, color, religion, gender, pregnancy, or national origin. In general, Title VII applies to employers with 15 or more employees. The purpose of the Title VII protections is to "level the playing field" by forcing employers to consider only objective, job-related criteria in making employment decisions. The preceding classes of individuals are considered "protected" under Title VII because of the history of unequal treatment that has been identified in each class. Title VII must be considered when employers review applications or resumes (i.e., by not eliminating candidates on the basis of a "foreign" last name), interview candidates (i.e., by asking only job-related questions), test job applicants (i.e., by treating all candidates the same and ensuring that tests are not unfairly weighted against any group of people), and consider employees for promotions, transfers, or any other employment-related benefit or condition.

The Civil Rights Act of 1991

The Civil Rights Act of 1964 was amended in 1991 to strengthen and improve federal civil rights laws, to provide for damages in cases of intentional employment discrimination, to clarify provisions regarding disparate impact actions, and for other purposes.

Sexual harassment. Sexual harassment is a form of sex discrimination that may violate Title VII of the Civil Rights Act. Title VII applies to all employers with 15 or more employees, including public sector organizations. It also applies to employment agencies, labor organizations, and the federal government.

Unwelcome sexual advances, requests for sexual favors, and other verbal or physical conduct of a sexual nature constitute sexual harassment when this conduct explicitly or implicitly affects an individual's employment, unreasonably interferes with an individual's work performance, or creates an intimidating, hostile, or offensive work environment.

Sexual harassment may occur in a variety of circumstances, including but not limited to the following:

- The victim as well as the harasser may be a woman or a man. The victim does not have to be of the opposite sex.

53

- The harasser can be the victim's supervisor, an agent of the employer, a supervisor in another area, a co-worker, or a nonemployee.
- The victim does not have to be the person harassed, but could be anyone affected by the offensive conduct.
- Unlawful sexual harassment may occur without economic injury to or discharge of the victim.
- The harasser's conduct must be unwelcome.

Age Discrimination in Employment Act

The Age Discrimination in Employment Act of 1967 (ADEA) protects individuals who are 40 years of age or older from employment discrimination based on age. The ADEA's protections apply to both employees and job applicants. Under the ADEA, it is unlawful to discriminate against a person because of his or her age with respect to any term, condition, or privilege of employment, including hiring, firing, promotion, layoff, compensation, benefits, job assignments, and training.

Americans with Disabilities Act

The Americans with Disabilities Act (ADA) is a federal antidiscrimination law that prohibits private employers, state and local governments, employment agencies, and labor unions from discriminating against qualified individuals with disabilities in job application procedures, hiring, firing, advancement, compensation, job training, and other terms, conditions, and privileges of employment. This law (covering employers with 15 or more employees) is designed to remove barriers that prevent qualified individuals with disabilities from enjoying the same employment opportunities that are available to persons without disabilities. When an individual's disability creates a barrier to employment opportunities, the ADA requires employers to consider whether a reasonable accommodation could remove the barrier.

Consolidated Omnibus Budget Reconciliation Act

The Consolidated Omnibus Budget Reconciliation Act (COBRA) gives workers and their families who lose their health benefits the right to choose to continue group health benefits provided by their group health plan for limited periods of time under certain circumstances such as voluntary or involuntary job loss, reduction in the hours worked, transition between jobs, death, divorce, and other life events. Qualified individuals may be required to pay the entire premium for coverage up to 102 percent of the cost to the plan.

The Consumer Credit Protection Plan

The federal wage garnishment law, Consumer Credit Protection Act (CCPA), protects employees from discharge by their employers because their wages have been garnished for any one debt, and limits the amount of an employee's earnings that may be garnished in any one week. The Wage and Hour Division (WHD) of the Department of Labor's (DOL) Employment Standards Administration (ESA) administers this act.

Drug-Free Workplace Act of 1988

The Drug-Free Workplace Act of 1988 requires some federal contractors and all federal grantees to agree that they will provide drug-free workplaces as a precondition of receiving a contract or grant from a federal agency.

Electronic Communications Privacy Act

The Electronic Communications Privacy Act (ECPA) sets out the provisions for access, use, disclosure, interception, and privacy protections of electronic communications. The law was enacted in 1986 and covers various forms of wire and electronic communications.

According to the U.S. Code, electronic communications "means any transfer of signs, signals, writing, images, sounds, data, or intelligence of any nature transmitted in whole or in part by a wire, radio, electromagnetic, photo electronic or photo optical system that affects interstate or foreign commerce." ECPA prohibits unlawful access and certain disclosures of communication contents. Additionally, the law prevents government entities from requiring disclosure of electronic communications from a provider without proper procedure.

The Employee Polygraph Protection Act

The Employee Polygraph Protection Act of 1988 (EPPA) generally prevents employers from using lie detector tests, either for preemployment screening or during the course of employment, with certain exemptions. Employers generally may not require or request any employee or job applicant to take a lie detector test, or discharge, discipline, or discriminate against an employee or job applicant for refusing to take a test or for exercising other rights under the act. In addition, employers are required to display the EPPA poster in the workplace for their employees.

Employee Retirement Income Security Act

The Employee Retirement Income Security Act of 1974 (ERISA) is a federal law that sets minimum standards for most voluntarily established pension and health plans in private industry to provide protection for individuals in these plans.

The Equal Pay Act of 1963

No employer shall discriminate, within any establishment in which such employees are employed, between employees on the basis of sex by paying wages to employees in such establishment at a rate less than the rate at which the employer pays wages to employees of the opposite sex in such establishment for equal work on jobs the performance of which requires equal skill, effort, and responsibility, and which are performed under similar working conditions, except where such payment is made pursuant to (1) a seniority system; (2) a merit system; (3) a system that measures earnings by quantity or quality of production; or (4) a differential based on any other factor other than sex. An employer who is paying a wage rate differential in violation of this act shall not reduce the wage rate of any employee to comply with the provisions of this act.

Executive Order 11246—Affirmative Action

This executive order prohibits federal contractors from discriminating against employees on the basis of race, color, religion, gender, or national origin. It is similar to the Civil Rights Act, but has the further requirement that federal contractors with contracts exceeding $50,000 and a workforce of more than 50 employees maintain an Affirmative Action Plan regarding the utilization of people in the protected classes.

Fair Credit Reporting Act

Employers who have a business need to evaluate and monitor employee credit problems and who use credit reports to do so should also be aware of the Fair Credit Reporting Act (FCRA). The FCRA requires employers who deny employment on the basis of a credit report to so notify the applicant and to provide the name and address of the consumer reporting agency used.

Fair Labor Standards Act

The Fair Labor Standards Act (FLSA) establishes minimum wage, overtime pay, recordkeeping, and child labor standards affecting full-time and part-time workers in the private sector and in federal, state, and local governments. Covered nonexempt workers are entitled to a minimum wage of not less than $5.15 an hour. (*Editor's note: The minimum wage shown here was accurate when this book was published, however, Congress could increase the amount at any time.*) Overtime pay at a rate of not less than one and one-half times their regular rates of pay is required after 40 hours of work in a workweek.

The Family and Medical Leave Act

The Family and Medical Leave Act (FMLA) allows employees who have met minimum service requirements (12 months employed by the company with 1,250 hours of service in the preceding 12 months) to take up to 12 weeks of unpaid leave (1) for a serious health condition, (2) to care for a family member with a serious health condition, (3) for the birth of a child, or (4) for the placement of a child for adoption or foster care.

Health Plans and Benefits

Portability of Health Coverage

The Health Insurance Portability and Accountability Act (HIPAA) provides rights and protections for participants and beneficiaries in group health plans. HIPAA includes protections for coverage under group health plans that limit exclusions for preexisting conditions, prohibit discrimination against employees and dependants based on their health status, and allow a special opportunity to enroll in a new plan to individuals in certain circumstances. HIPAA may also give you a right to purchase individual coverage if you have no group health plan coverage available and have exhausted COBRA or other continuation coverage.

Mental Health Act

The Mental Health Parity Act of 1996 (MHPA) prohibits group health plans and insurance companies that offer mental health benefits from setting annual or lifetime limits on mental health benefits that are lower than those limits set for any other condition. For example, if a plan does not impose an annual or lifetime limit on benefits paid out for surgery, it cannot impose limits on mental health benefits. The MHPA requirements apply to group health plans for plan years beginning on or after January 1, 1998, through September 31, 2001. There are two exemptions to this law. It does not apply to small employers (2 to 50 employees) or to group health plans whose costs would increase 1 percent or more as a result of compliance.

Newborns' and Mothers' Health Protection Act

The Newborns' and Mothers' Health Protection Act of 1996 (NMHPA) requires a minimum length of hospital confinement in conjunction with childbirth. This requirement applies to health plans and health insurance companies that provide hospital stays for childbirth in their policies. The law provides that coverage for a hospital stay following a normal delivery may not be limited to less than 48 hours for both the mother and newborn, and for a cesarean section not less than 96 hours. This law also prevents plans from charging greater deductibles, coinsurance, or other cost-sharing measures for benefits relating to hospital stays for childbirth. The NMHPA requirements apply to group health plans for plan years beginning on or after January 1, 1998.

The Immigration and Nationality Act

The Immigration and Nationality Act (INA) sets forth the conditions for the temporary and permanent employment of aliens in the United States and includes provisions that address employment eligibility and employment verification. These provisions apply to all employers.

This act describes what employers must do to verify the identity and employment eligibility of anyone to be hired and the protections afforded to employees from discrimination in hiring or discharge on the basis of national origin and citizenship status.

Immigration Reform and Control Act

The Immigration Reform and Control Act (IRCA) prohibits the employment of individuals who are not legally authorized to work in the United States or in an employment classification that they are not authorized to fill. The IRCA requires employers to certify (using the I-9 form) within three days of employment the identity and eligibility to work of all employees hired. I-9 forms must be retained for three years following employment or one year following termination, whichever is later.

The IRCA also prohibits discrimination in employment-related matters on the basis of national origin or citizenship. Discriminatory actions include, but are not limited to, requesting additional documents beyond those required, refusing to accept valid documents or consider an applicant who is suspected of being an illegal alien, or harassing or retaliating against employees for exercising their rights under the law.

Labor Management Relations Act

Taft-Hartley Labor Act

Taft-Hartley Labor Act, 1947, passed by the U.S. Congress, is officially known as the Labor-Management Relations Act. The act qualified or amended much of the National Labor Relations (Wagner) Act of 1935, the federal law regulating labor relations of enterprises engaged in interstate commerce. The act establishes control of labor disputes on a new basis by enlarging the National Labor Relations Board and providing that the union or the employer must, before terminating a collective-bargaining agreement, serve notice on the other party and on a government mediation service. The act also prohibits jurisdictional strikes (disputes between two unions

over which should act as the bargaining agent for the employees) and secondary boycotts (boycotts against an already organized company doing business with another company that a union is trying to organize), declares that it did not extend protection to workers on wildcat strikes, outlaws the closed shop, and permits the union shop only on a vote of a majority of the employees. The act also forbids unions to contribute to political campaigns.

National Labor Relations Act

The National Labor Relations Act (NLRA), passed in 1935, provides that all employees have the right to form, join, and assist labor organizations and to bargain collectively with their employers. The National Labor Relations Board enforces the act, and the body of decisions and regulations from the board has formed an extensive set of standards for electing and decertifying unions, for negotiating bargaining agreements, and for defining activities as fair or unfair labor practices.

Occupational Safety and Health Act

The Occupational Safety and Health Act of 1970 (OSHA) includes a "general duty clause" that requires virtually all employers to maintain a workplace that is free from recognized hazards that would cause injury or death to employees. Most employers must comply with OSHA workplace safety and health standards that apply to their workplaces. OSHA requires employers to maintain a log of certain injuries and illnesses, report certain deaths and multiple hospitalizations, and post supplementary records on an annual basis. Employers may not discharge employees who refuse to do a job that, by their reasonable apprehension, places them at risk of injury or exposes them to a hazardous workplace condition. The standards are voluminous and may be obtained from the Government Printing Office.

Older Workers Benefit Protection Act

The Older Workers Benefit Protection Act of 1990 (OWBPA) amended the ADEA to specifically prohibit employers from denying benefits to older employees. An employer may reduce benefits based on age only if the cost of providing the reduced benefits to older workers is the same as the cost of providing benefits to younger workers.

Uniformed Services Employment and Reemployment Rights Act

The Uniformed Services Employment and Reemployment Rights Act (USERRA), which replaces the Veterans' Reemployment Rights Act, very broadly prohibits employers from discriminating against individuals because of past, present, or future membership in a uniformed service (including periods of voluntary training and service). The act (1) prohibits discrimination in employment, job retention, and advancement; (2) requires employers to provide retraining opportunities; (3) requires healthcare and pension benefits to continue during leave; (4) allows an employee to take military leave up to five years; (5) provides additional protection for disabled veterans; (6) requires employees to provide notice of their need for leave; and (7) requires service members to notify their employers of their intention to return to work. Individuals reemployed after a period of military service are generally required to be allowed to return to work to all the benefits and seniority they would have had if they had remained continuously employed.

Pregnancy Discrimination Act

The Pregnancy Discrimination Act is an amendment to Title VII of the Civil Rights Act of 1964. Discrimination on the basis of pregnancy, childbirth, or related medical conditions constitutes unlawful sex discrimination under Title VII. Women affected by pregnancy or related conditions must be treated in the same manner as other applicants or employees with similar abilities or limitations.

The Personal Responsibility and Work Opportunity Reconciliation Act

The Personal Responsibility and Work Opportunity Reconciliation Act of 1996 requires work in exchange for time-limited assistance. The bill contains strong work requirements, a performance bonus to reward states for moving welfare recipients into jobs, state maintenance of effort requirements, comprehensive child support enforcement, and supports for families moving from welfare to work, including increased funding for child care and guaranteed medical coverage.

Vietnam Era Veterans' Readjustment Assistance Act

The Vietnam Era Veterans' Readjustment Assistance Act of 1974 (VEVRAA) requires that employers with federal contracts or subcontracts of $25,000 or more provide equal opportunity and affirmative action for Vietnam-era veterans, special disabled veterans, and veterans who served on active duty during a war or in a campaign or expedition for which a campaign badge has been authorized.

The Rehabilitation Act of 1973, Section 503

Section 503 of the Rehabilitation Act of 1973 prohibits discrimination and requires employers with federal contracts or subcontracts that exceed $10,000 to take affirmative action to hire, retain, and promote qualified individuals with disabilities. All covered contractors and subcontractors must also include a specific equal opportunity clause in each of their nonexempt contracts and subcontracts.

GLOSSARY

Achievement test: A selection tool used to measure current knowledge or skills.

Acuity: Acuteness, as of an illness. The greater the acuity, the more nursing care or other services are needed. (*Slee's Health Care Terms, Third Comprehensive Edition*)

Adverse impact: A method of proving discrimination reflecting an applicant rejection rate for a protected class that is higher than the rate for the unprotected class.

Affirmative Action: A remedy for past discrimination that increases the numbers of protected classes in the organization's workforce.

Americans with Disabilities Act (ADA): Federal legislation that makes it illegal to discriminate against people with disabilities in employment decisions.

Apprenticeship: An on-the-job training technique used in the skilled trades to allow an inexperienced employee to learn the craft from a skilled worker.

Aptitude test: A selection tool used to measure the applicant's capacity to learn new skills.

Behaviorally Anchored Rating Scale (BARS): A performance appraisal system that uses scales anchored by descriptions of critical incidents to measure behaviors of employees on the job.

Bona Fide Occupational Qualification (BFOQ): A legal exception to discrimination whereby the employer may specify hiring based on gender, age, religion, sex, or national origin.

Broadbanding: A compensation system that collapses several salary grades into a few broader categories.

Cognitive ability test: A selection test used to measure mental skills.

Comparable worth: The equality of jobs performed by women and men in terms of the value or worth to the company (though the jobs are different).

E-commerce: Conducting business over the Internet.

Elder care: Care provided to elderly family members of an employee.

Employee assistance programs (EAPs): Services provided to employees to counsel and advise for problems interfering with work performance.

Employee involvement groups: Groups of employees who meet to resolve specific problems in the organization.

Employee leasing: Hiring employees back through leasing companies to perform their original function.

Employment-at-will: The right of an employer and an employee to terminate the employment relationship without reason.

Empowerment: Delegating power throughout the organization to encourage employees to make decisions concerning their own work.

Equal employment opportunity: The treatment of employees in a fair and impartial way in all aspects of employment.

Equity theory: A social comparison motivation theory in which people compare the ratio of their inputs to outputs to the ratio of another person's inputs to outputs.

Ergonomics: The study of the design of equipment in the workplace. Equipment is fit to people to reduce the possibility of injuries.

Ethics: Individual beliefs concerning right and wrong.

Eustress: Positive stress that propels people to higher levels of performance.

Expatriate managers: Managers in multinational corporations sent on international assignments from their home country.

Hierarchy of needs: Motivation theory developed by Abraham Maslow to explain the needs that drive people's behavior.

Hostile environment: Harassment that results from the creation of an offensive work environment.

Human relations skills: Interpersonal skills.

Human resource management: The set of activities focused on the effective management and development of the organization's workforce.

Human resource planning (HRP): The process of identifying the future staffing needs of the organization.

Human resources: The people of the organization.

Human Resources Information System (HRIS): A computer system designed to aid in the administration and decision-making process of human resource management.

Integrity tests: Paper and pencil tests to measure honesty in the selection process.

Job analysis: The process of systematically gathering information concerning the tasks and responsibilities of a job.

Job characteristics model: An approach to job design that results in increased performance levels and greater worker motivation.

Job description: A document that itemizes the tasks and responsibilities of a job.

Job design: A method of structuring jobs to improve worker satisfaction and organizational performance.

Job enlargement: A job design technique that expands a job by adding tasks that are on the same responsibility level.

Job enrichment: A job design technique that adds tasks on a higher responsibility level to increase job satisfaction.

On-the-job training: Training provided in a hands-on approach.

Orientation: The socialization process that is used to acquaint employees with the organization.

Outplacement: Services offered to help employees who have been terminated find new employment.

Outsourcing: Contracting with outside firms to perform nonessential functions for the organization.

Part-time employees: Those employees who work fewer than 40 hours a week.

Pay equity: The perception of employees that their compensation is equal to the worth of their work.

Pay secrecy: The extent to which an organization keeps individual pay rates a secret.

Peer appraisal: Performance appraisals performed by co-workers.

Performance appraisal: The formal evaluation of an employee's work on the job.

Point system: A quantitative job evaluation system that uses specific elements of jobs to rate their worth to the organization.

Progressive discipline: The method of discipline that uses a system of progressively more serious punishments for violations.

Protected classes: Women, people with disabilities, minority races, and older people in the workforce.

Punishment: Unpleasant consequences resulting from specific behaviors.

Quid pro quo harassment: Harassment that occurs with an exchange of sexual favors for employment decisions.

Realistic job preview (RJP): A realistic portrayal of a job that includes both its negative and positive aspects.

Stress: The emotional and physical wear and tear of life.

Structured interview: An interview conducted with job applicants using prepared questions.

Succession planning: The process of identifying and tracking potential management candidates.

Telecommuting: The use of computer technology to work from home or satellite offices via electronic links to the office.

Temporary employees: Workers who are employed for specific periods and who are not permanent employees of the firm.

Title VII of the Civil Rights Act: Federal legislation that prohibits discrimination in all employment decisions based on race, religion, color, sex, or national origin.

Transfer of training: The application of training material to job performance.

Trend analysis: A quantitative forecasting technique used to identify the demand for labor.

Unemployment insurance: A required benefit that provides income to employees who are out of work.

Vestibule training: Simulation training that mirrors actual job conditions.

Virtual team: A team that works together from different geographic locations using electronic links.

Wellness programs: Organizational programs that emphasize keeping workers healthy.

Workers' compensation insurance: Insurance payments made to employees who suffer illnesses or injuries on the job.

Yield ratio: A calculation of the percentage of job candidates from a specific recruitment source who make it to the next stage of the selection process.

PRACTICE QUESTIONS

1. The immigration Form I-9 must be completed:
   A. upon hire of all employees.
   B. upon hire of all foreign employees.
   C. within 3 days on all employees.
   D. within 3 days on all foreign employees.

   A B C D
   ○ ○ ○ ○

2. The ability of an employer to terminate an employee without cause is recognized in most states; what is this is called?
   A. Contract employee
   B. Implied contract
   C. Oral contract
   D. At-will doctrine

   A B C D
   ○ ○ ○ ○

3. What is the greatest operational challenge most assisted living residences will encounter?
   A. Insufficient seniors to maintain occupancy
   B. Changes in state and federal laws
   C. Recruitment and retention of staff
   D. Maintaining continued profitability.

   A B C D
   ○ ○ ○ ○

4. What is the first thing you should do before hiring a new employee?
   A. Interview the candidates for the job
   B. Have a job description for position
   C. Advertise the job in local papers
   D. Write the contract to be offered

   A B C D
   ○ ○ ○ ○

5. The most efficacious way to recruit staff is through:
   A. job fairs.
   B. existing employees.
   C. newspaper/publications.
   D. the Internet.

   A B C D
   ○ ○ ○ ○

6. The next major demographic population we must prepare for is referred to as the:
   A. Baby Boomers.
   B. Millennials.
   C. Generation Xers.
   D. "Now" Generation.

   A B C D
   ○ ○ ○ ○

7. All but which one of the following is commonly accepted as an intended purpose of the annual performance evaluations?
   A. Determine pay increase
   B. Confirm nationality and marital status
   C. Review performance of the job
   D. Act as a communication tool

   A B C D
   ○ ○ ○ ○

8. What is one of the most important and overlooked investments an RC/AL facility makes?
   A. Sufficient parking for staff and visitors
   B. Orientation and training of staff
   C. Security systems
   D. Emergency generators

   A B C D
   ○ ○ ○ ○

9. Medical exams, toxic substance exposure records, and blood-borne pathogen exposure records must be kept for how long?
   A. 1 year
   B. 5 years
   C. 15 years
   D. 30 years

   A B C D
   ○ ○ ○ ○

10. One qualification of FLMA is that an employee must have worked a minimum of 1250 hours:
   A. after probationary period.
   B. since date of hire.
   C. over the past 12 months.
   D. in a calendar year.

   A B C D
   ○ ○ ○ ○

ANSWERS AND EXPLANATIONS

1. **Correct answer = D.** All employees must complete Form I-9 within three days of employment.
2. **Correct answer = D.** The at-will doctrine states that an employee is employed at the will of his or her employer who has the right to terminate without cause.
3. **Correct answer = C.** The shrinking workforce and high rate of retirement are creating the greatest set of challenges assisted living will face now and in the future.
4. **Correct answer = B.** Without a job description, neither you nor the employee can establish clear job requirements and expectations.
5. **Correct answer = B.** Word of mouth will always be the most effective and efficient way to recruit new employees.
6. **Correct answer = B.** The Millennials are quickly becoming the largest segment of the workforce, and this development will require a new understanding of their social and work characteristics to know how to lead them effectively.
7. **Correct answer = B.** Nationality and marital status are not factors that should enter into hiring arrangements or ongoing performance appraisals.
8. **Correct answer = B.** Orientation and training of staff establish the preparation and understanding of your staff in executing their job responsibilities, as well as your mutual understanding of each other's job expectations.
9. **Correct answer = D.** All of the records cited must be maintained for a minimum of 30 years.
10. **Correct answer = C.** According to federal law, an employee must have first been employed for 12 months and worked an average of at least 1,250 hours during that 12-month period.

REFERENCES

Adams, Bob. 1996. *Small Business Start-Up.* F & W Publications Company.

Buhler, Patricia. 2002. *Human Resources Management.* Streetwise Publications.

Elliott, Robert. 1998. *Human Resource Management, Residential Care/Assisted Living Administrator's Exam Study Guide.* Washington, DC: National Association of Boards of Examiners of Long Term Care Administrators.

Fleischer, Charles H. 2005. *HR for Small Business.* Sphinx Publishing.

Grensing-Pophal, Lin. 2005. *Employee Management for Small Business.* International Self-Counsel Press.

Grote, Dick. 2002. *The Performance Appraisal Question and Answer Book.* American Management Association.

Harvard Business School Press. 2005. *Retaining Your Best People.* The Results Driven Manager Series. Harvard Business School Press.

Information Outlook. 2006. *Profile: The Hay Guide Chart Method of Job Evaluation.*

Losey, Meisinger, and Ulrich. *The Future of Human Resource Management.* New York: John Wiley.

Nelson, Bob. 1994. *1001 Ways to Reward Employees.* Workman Press.

Raines, Claire. 2003. *Connecting Generations: The Sourcebook for a New Workplace.* Crisp Publications.

Reichheld, Frederich. 1996. *The Loyalty Effect.* Harvard Business School Press.

Steingold, Fred S. 2003. *The Employer's Legal Handbook.* Nolo Publishers.

IMPORTANT WEB SITES

- AOL Legal Department. http://www.legal.web.aol.com
- Infoplease. http://www.infoplease.com
- Internal Revenue Service. http://www.irs.gov
- MedLawPlus. http://www.medlawplus.com

- National Employment Law Project. http://www.nelp.com
- Society of Human Resources Management. http://www.shrm.org
- U.S. Department of Labor. http://www.dol.gov
- U.S. Department of Labor, Bureau of Labor Statistics. http://www.bls.gov
- U.S. Department of Labor, Employment and Training Administration. http://www.doleta.gov
- U.S. Equal Employment Opportunity Commission. http://www.eeoc.gov
- U.S. Social Security Administration. http://www.ssa.gov
- World at Work (benefits and compensation training organization). http://www.worldatwork.org

DIANE K. DUIN, PhD, MHA, LNHA, is the health scholar and assessment director for the Health Administration Program in the College of Allied Health Professions at Montana State University—Billings. She has a doctorate in rural sociology. Dr. Duin is a licensed nursing home administrator. She is a member of the American College of Healthcare Executives (ACHE); the Gerontological Society of America; and the American Corrections Association. She has served as a member of the editorial board for the ACHE Management Series, a member of the South Dakota ACHE Regent's Advisory Council, and on the board of directors for Sioux Valley Vermillion Medical Center in Vermillion, South Dakota. Dr. Duin has served as the director of a long term care management certificate program. Additionally, she has written articles and cases on gerontology, long term care education, demographic changes, and healthcare reform.

CHAPTER 5

LEADERSHIP AND GOVERNANCE

Diane K. Duin, PhD, MHA, LNHA

Introduction

The rapid expansion of residential care and assisted living (RC/AL) facilities in the United States presents current and aspiring **administrators** with a variety of challenges and opportunities. The scope of an administrator's responsibilities begins with understanding the philosophy of assisted living and residential care. Although these services are a significant piece in the long term care continuum, a common definition for RC/AL services does not exist. Each state regulates and monitors facilities according to the individual state. RC/AL residences offer a wide range of personal and professional services that provide comfortable living for independent persons not wanting or able to live in their own home. These services are offered on both a scheduled and unscheduled basis 24 hours per day seven days per week. Because of this diversity in the provision and regulation of services, the overarching philosophy of RC/AL facilities focuses on person-centered care delivered within a hospitality model of service delivery.

In assisted living facilities, hospitality begins with the right attitude and is then delivered through the manager's leadership by example. The challenge for the RC/AL manager is to communicate to employees the importance of showing strong customer sensitivity and awareness through employing good listening skills (Wuenschel, in Namazi and Chafetz 2001).

In an October 2006 survey by MyInnerView, it was shown that leadership plays a vital role in shaping organizational culture and driving performance of long term care facilities. Researchers found that there were five leadership attributes that drive organizational performance: a focused visionary, strategic management, caring leadership, **communication**, and supporting change (Grant, Gulsvig, and Call 2006). Leaders of RC/AL organizations are key in setting the agenda and strategic direction of the facility, managing and motivating personnel, providing critical community connections and relationships, managing problems, and ensuring that systems are in place to achieve quality outcomes.

Regulation of Assisted Living

Federal laws affect assisted living, but assisted living is not defined or regulated by the federal government. State and local governments regulate the varying laws and **regulations** that affect assisted living. Regulations vary from state to state, and as a result, competition in the assisted living environment is often based on costs or charges, quality of service, level of service, and **staffing**.

Governance of Assisted Living

Different types of corporate structures may govern RC/AL facilities. They may be freestanding, **for-profit** companies or part of a larger chain of assisted living facilities. In these instances, their mission is to provide services and make a profit for their owners or outside investors, sometimes referred to as shareholders. Organizations can also be **not-for-profit** and may have an affiliation with a larger healthcare system or a religious denomination. In these cases, the facility's mission is to serve their stakeholders, and so the needs of the residents may take priority over making a financial return. Any financial losses of these organizations may be subsidized by philanthropy or the reserves of the parent organization.

If a limited liability partnership, a **corporation**, or political subdivision operates the RC/AL facility, there must be an organized governing body that is legally responsible for the overall conduct of the facility. The governing body develops the mission and vision and establishes and maintains administrative policies, procedures, or bylaws governing the operation of the facility. The governing body, or **board of directors**, normally hires the administrator and delegates the day-to-day **management** of the facility to the administrator. The governing body retains the ultimate responsibility for the well-being of the facility. This includes hiring and evaluating the administrator, fiduciary responsibility, and financial viability. If an individual or **partnership** operates the RC/AL, the individual or partnership establishes the administrative policies, procedures, or bylaws for the operation of the facility. In some RC/AL facilities, a community **advisory board** may be used to provide guidance to the administrator regarding appropriate **policies** and **procedures** for administration of the facility.

The Administrator as Leader

Leadership Styles

Leadership is the process of **influencing** people while meeting organizational requirements. Leadership has been conceptualized in many ways; however, four components are necessary for leadership to occur. First, leadership is a process. It is interactive in nature. Second, leadership involves influencing others. Third, leadership occurs in groups. One cannot be a leader without followers. Finally, leadership involves attaining **goals**. This means that leadership has to do with **directing** a group toward accomplishing goals (Northouse 2004).

There are a number of leadership theories and styles. Leadership style is the manner and approach of providing direction, implementing plans, and motivating people. There are three common styles of leadership:

- Authoritarian or autocratic
- **Participative** or democratic
- **Laissez-faire** or free reign

Authoritarian or autocratic. This style is used when the leader tells his or her employees what he or she wants done and how it is to be done, without getting the advice of the employee. Some of the appropriate conditions to use authoritarian or autocratic leadership are when the leader has all the information to solve the problem, is short on time, and the employees are well motivated.

Participative or democratic. This type of style involves the leader including one or more employees in the decision-making process (determining what to do and how to do it). However, the leader maintains the final decision-making authority. Using this style is not a sign of weakness; rather it is a sign of strength that employees will respect (McConnell 2006).

Participative or democratic leadership is normally used when the leader has part of the information, and the employees have the other parts. A leader is not expected to know everything—this is why the leader employs knowledgeable and skillful employees. Using this style of leadership is of mutual benefit; it allows the employees to become part of the team and allows the leader to make better decisions.

Laissez-faire or free reign. In this style, the leader allows the employees to make the decision. However, the leader is still responsible for the decisions that are made. Laissez-faire or free reign is used when employees are able to analyze the situation and determine what needs to be done and how to do it. This style is best used when the leader has full trust and confidence in the people below him or her. Laissez-faire can be effective with motivated and knowledgeable employees and with professional staff (Northouse 2004).

Leadership and Management

Leadership and *management* are terms that are frequently confused by those who are unfamiliar with what each means. This section defines management and its function and leadership in the RC/AL facility.

Leaders can be managers, but managers are not always leaders. A manager is in charge because of an official designation. Managers get things done through and with other people. Management and leadership can be very similar, but at the same time, they are different. A manager in the RC/AL facility is a person who takes responsibility to ensure that the goals of the facility are met. Managers are appointed but never emergent.

A leader may be appointed, but he or she may also be an emergent leader, someone who had no intention of leading. A leader inspires others to move the facility forward. A leader is visionary. Management and leadership share some characteristics, but they can also be very different.

Management, or a manager, directs and controls the day-to-day functions of the facility. The manager directs of the work of employees and is responsible for results. Managers must make sure that the everyday events that need to take place actually do take place. Managers also handle disciplinary actions and employee concerns that may arise.

On the other hand, leadership is not necessarily involved in day-to-day operations. Leadership is a powerful driver to achieving organizational excellence and obtaining quality service outcomes. The administrator of an RC/AL facility is a leader and can inspire employees with a vision for the facility and help them cope with change. Leaders make people want to achieve the goals of the organization. Leadership involves inspiring and motivating individuals. People tend to "follow" leaders because the leader is respected. In management, employees under the manager do what they need to do because it is their job. It is much more difficult to be a leader than it is to be a manager because of the fact that leaders must gain the respect of individuals.

Leadership drives performance through its influence on organizational culture. Leadership sets the agenda, supports change, and enhances communication (Grant et al. 2006). Being an effective administrator requires an understanding of both leadership and the functions of management. Without understanding how management works, leadership will become ineffective, and the quality agenda of the RC/AL facility will not be achieved.

Functions of Management

Traditionally, the term *management* refers to the activities of **planning**, decision making, **organizing**, staffing, directing, and **controlling**. These management functions are tools that the administrator uses to achieve organizational effectiveness.

Planning

Planning is defined as "the process of deciding in the present what to do to bring about an outcome in the future" (Liebler 2005, 83). The problem with planning is that it involves circumstances, events, people, and actions that cannot be predicted. Therefore, planning is a tentative process.

To plan for an organization requires many phases. It requires that the organization clarify its mission, values, and vision. A **mission statement** defines the organization's purpose. A **vision statement** describes the desired future position for the organization. Values include the principles by which the organization guides its overall actions. The organization's sponsor or **governance** body

69

most often directs the mission, vision and values of an RC/AL facility.

Some senior administrators write the organization's overall mission and vision statements. Other managers at different levels may write mission statements for their particular divisions or departments, but ones that are consistent with the wider mission, vision, and values of the organization. The mission statement development process requires administrators to do the following:

- Clearly identify the organization's culture, values, strategy, and view of the future.
- Address the commitment the organization has to its stakeholders.
- Ensure that the objectives are measurable, the approach is actionable, and the vision is achievable.
- Communicate the message.
- Develop support throughout the organization.

Mission and vision statements are used in the following ways:

- Internally:
  - Guide the thinking of management with respect to strategic issues.
  - Help define performance standards.
  - Focus on common goals, inspire employees.
  - Guide decision making throughout the organization.
  - Establish a framework for ethical behavior.
- Externally:
  - Enlist external support.
  - Create closer linkages and better communication with stakeholders.
  - Serve as a marketing tool.

The goals and objectives for the facility and the departments within the facility are more explicit than the mission statement is. Goals are statements that specify what should be accomplished by the facility or department. Goals are written that are specific, measurable, realistic and have a timeline. Objectives

or tactics specify what is to be done, how much is to be done, and by when it is to be done. Objectives are measurable and time-specific. Action steps are very specific as to what will be done to accomplish the goals and objectives.

Policies and procedures provide employees with guides for their actions. A policy is an expression of what and why, and a procedure describes how.

The final element is evaluation. Each of these phases of planning must be evaluated to determine effectiveness. The administrator and governing board review vision and mission statements on a regular basis. Because they are the core purpose and targeted future of the facility, it is generally believed that mission statements are written in such a fashion so as not to require frequent review. If a facility changes the way it does business, or through whom it is affiliated to do business, or the business, regulatory, or economic environment changes, the facility should evaluate its vision and mission statement.

Goals and objectives should be evaluated at least on an annual basis. Objectives should be evaluated more frequently because they are measurable and time-specific. When goals and objectives are evaluated, there may be a change in the action plans. Formal (yearly department planning sessions) and informal (when objectives are reached) evaluations may be done. The purpose of evaluating plans is to provide **feedback** and adjust planning to reflect any changes that may have occurred.

The RC/AL facility's **strategic planning** process is the responsibility of the administrator in conjunction with the facility's stakeholders, typically the governance organization. Stakeholders are those individuals or organizations that have an interest in the RC/AL facility and its success. Although many individuals or organizations may be stakeholders, examples include a vendor, an employee, or a resident. The facility's strategic planning process involves evaluating the mission statement of the facility. Strategic planning requires the administrator to work with the stakeholders to determine the appropriate allocation of resources to carry out the goals and objectives established to serve the mission of the facility.

The strategic planning process also involves creating the long-range vision for the facility. The vision, a statement of the desired future of the facility, guides the administrator and the stakeholders in prioritizing the objectives for the facility.

When the strategic planning process is complete, it is essential that the administrator clearly define and communicate the organization's vision and objectives to its stakeholders. Employees should be involved in working to establish objectives within the facility. The objectives established by the facility's employees must be consistent with the vision, mission, and objectives established for the overall facility. The key to ensuring the success of the planning process is for the administrator to make certain everyone involved with the facility is aligned in creating the desired future of the facility.

Organizing

Authority versus responsibility. **Authority** refers to the formal or official power of the administrator to obtain the compliance of those working with him or her by using directives, communications, policies, and objectives. Authority is associated with the administrator's function in the organization. The authority is actually vested in organizational roles or positions. As long as an individual holds the position, he or she has the privilege of exercising the authority of the position.

Responsibility is the obligation of the employee to perform the duty as assigned. By accepting a job and accepting the obligation to perform the assigned tasks affiliated with the job, an employee accepts responsibility. From the administrator's perspective responsibility cannot be delegated. The administrator can assign a task and delegate the authority to perform a specific job to an employee; however, the administrator does not delegate responsibility for accomplishment of the task.

Span of management. **Span of management** is the number of people any one person supervises effectively. There is no ideal number for span of management. At the upper levels of administration, there are fewer subordinate managers reporting to an upper-level administrator. As one moves down the managerial hierarchy, the span of management generally increases. It is not uncommon for a midlevel manager to have 15 to 20 people reporting to him or her.

The number of people one can effectively supervise depends on a number of different factors, such as frequency of contact with others and the intensity of the contact with others. Before determining an actual number for the span of management, it is necessary to examine the factors involved in each of the contacts.

Line and staff relationships. The difference between line and staff is frequently confused. Some of the confusion comes from the informal meaning of *staff*, which is generally considered as the grouping of individuals who perform a similar task in different departments. In management theory, the term *staff* refers to an individual or individuals who serve in an advisory capacity to the administrator of an organization. Line personnel typically have direct responsibility to ensure goals are achieved through others (Dunn 2002). Frequently, on **organizational charts** the staff relationship is indicated by a dotted line. This dotted line is defined as providing an advisory function. A solid line on an organizational chart indicates direct reporting/responsibility between the two positions.

Organizational charts. Organizational charts are line drawings of the reporting relationships throughout the organization. Employees can see with ease to whom they are responsible. Figure 5.1 is a typical, simplified organizational chart.

71

Figure 5.1 An organizational chart.

.... Line relationship
———————————— Staff relationship

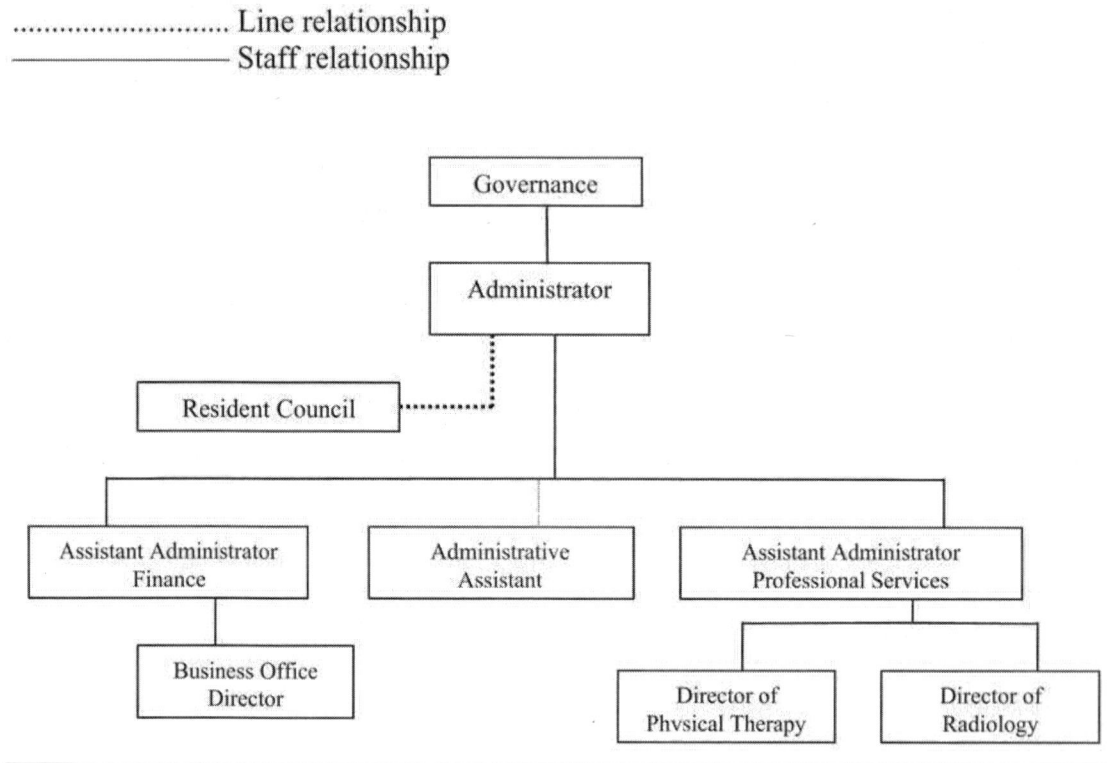

Job descriptions. **Job descriptions** provide an organization with information regarding how the work will be done. In every formal organization, a job description covers every job.

Staffing

Employees are the human resources of the RC/AL facility. Without employees, the facility would not be able to do the work that needs to be done. Administrators in the RC/AL facility are responsible for maintaining desired staffing levels by having a qualified and stable number of employees. Recruiting employees helps to build a qualified and stable workforce and provides opportunities for employees to improve their skills while ensuring employees are satisfied with their responsibilities and the work environment. The administrator needs to identify his or her staff requirements, clearly define the positions

through job descriptions, and develop systems to select, train, and retain staff.

Staff training and development. One of the primary goals of managing human resources should be an employee's personal development. Such development involves preparing individuals to function responsibly in the RC/AL facility. The programs of performance evaluation and training should be designed to promote this objective.

Decision Making

Making an effective decision requires an action. Making a decision implies that there are alternative choices to be considered even when one of the alternatives is to make no decision. The administrator not only wants to identify as many of these alternatives as possible, but also choose the one that best fits with the mission, values, and goals of the facility.

Very few decisions are made with absolute certainty because complete knowledge about all the alternatives is seldom possible. Thus, every decision involves a certain amount of risk.

Liebler and McConnell (2004) identify three steps in the decision process:

1. Agenda building—discuss and prioritize the issues.
2. Search for alternatives—list all of the possible alternatives you have for making the decision.
3. Evaluation of alternatives—select from the listed alternatives the best one for making the decision.

Problem solving and decision making are intertwined. There are many approaches to problem solving, depending on the type of problem and the people involved. The more traditional approach involves describing and clarifying the problem, analyzing its causes, identifying alternative solutions, assessing each alternative, choosing one, implementing it, and evaluating whether the problem was solved.

Controlling or Feedback

The management function of controlling is the feedback step. It establishes performance standards based on the firm's objectives, measures and reports performance relative to the organization's goals, compares the two, and takes corrective or preventive action as necessary. Controlling is concerned with making certain that work is properly executed. Controlling is closely related to all management functions, but it is most closely related to the planning function. As the administrator plans, he or she sets the direction, goals, and objectives and develops policies. The facility's performance is checked and evaluated against these standards.

The purpose of the controlling process is to ensure that performance is *consistent* with plans, that plans and standards are being adhered to, and that proper progress is being made toward objectives. Management is concerned with controls that anticipate potential sources of deviation from standards. Past experience and the study of past events tell the administrator what has taken place and where, when, and why certain standards were not met. This enables management to make provisions so that future activities will not lead to these deviations.

Strategies for control or process alignment. Benchmarking is a process alignment strategy. Benchmarking is establishing the values against which the administrator compares his or her facility or department with the level of activity or results of another facility or department. Benchmarking information may be available from consulting firms or industry association organizations. Benchmarking seeks best practices so that the facility remains competitive in the marketplace.

Tools for control or process alignment. Tools for controlling/process alignment include a variety of statistical and graphical tools such as flow charts, run charts, histograms, scatter grams, cause-effect charts, and quality control charts. Walter Shewhart, the pioneering statistician who developed statistical process control in the Bell Laboratories in the United States during the 1930s, originally developed the concept of the Plan-Do-Check-Act (PDCA) Cycle. It is often referred to as the Shewhart Cycle (Figure 5.2). The PDCA Cycle is used to coordinate the facility's continuous improvement efforts (Kelly 2003).

Budget. A budget is a written plan expressed in figures and numerical terms, primarily in dollars and cents, that projects revenue and expenses for a specified time. Budgeting is a planning function, but the administration of the budget is part of the controlling function. Budgets are preestablished standards to which operations are compared and, if necessary, adjusted by the exercise of control. The budget is a means of control insofar as it reflects the progress of the actual performance against the plan. The budget is another tool of control as well as a tool for planning.

Directing. Directing involves influencing behavior through motivation, communication, leadership, and discipline. The purpose of directing is to focus the behavior of others in the organization to accomplishing the mission and objectives.

Team Building

Team building occurs when a team comes together and directs the energy toward problem solving, task effectiveness, and maximizing the resources of each of the members to accomplish a goal or purpose. **Teams** may also play an important role in the process of problem solving to achieve quality outcomes for the facility. Team building works best when the following 12 conditions are met:

1. There is a high level of commitment and interdependence among team members.
2. The team leader has good people skills, is committed to developing a team approach, and allocates time to team-building activities.
3. Each team member is capable and willing to contribute information, skills, and experiences that provide an appropriate mix for achieving the team's purpose.
4. The team develops a climate in which people feel relaxed and are able to be direct and open in their communications.
5. Team members develop a mutual trust and respect for each other and believe that other team members have skills and capabilities to contribute to the team.
6. Both the team and individual members are prepared to take risks and are

allowed to develop their abilities and skills.
7. The team is clear about its important goals and establishes performance targets that cause stretching but are achievable.
8. Team member roles are defined, and effective ways to solve problems and communicate are developed and supported by all team members.
9. Team members know how to examine team and individual errors and weaknesses without making personal attacks, which enables the group to learn from its experiences.
10. Team efforts are devoted to the achievement of results, and team performance is frequently evaluated to see where improvements can be made.
11. The team has the capacity to create new ideas through group interaction and the influence of outside people.
12. Each member of the team trusts the others and is aware that he or she can influence the team agenda. (Francis and Young 1979)

Consensus Building

Consensus building is a strategy that involves everyone playing a role in the decision making of the team. For this to be successful, it is important to be open to compromise. Consensus produces a team agreement at the conclusion. The following is a consensus-building procedure developed by the Triton and Patterns Project.

1. Agree on the objectives of the task, expectation and rules
2. Define the problem or decision to be reached by consensus
3. Figure out what must be done to reach a solution and brainstorm solutions
4. Discuss pros and cons from a list of ideas
5. Adjust, compromise, fine tune so all agree

Figure 5.2 The Shewart Cycle.

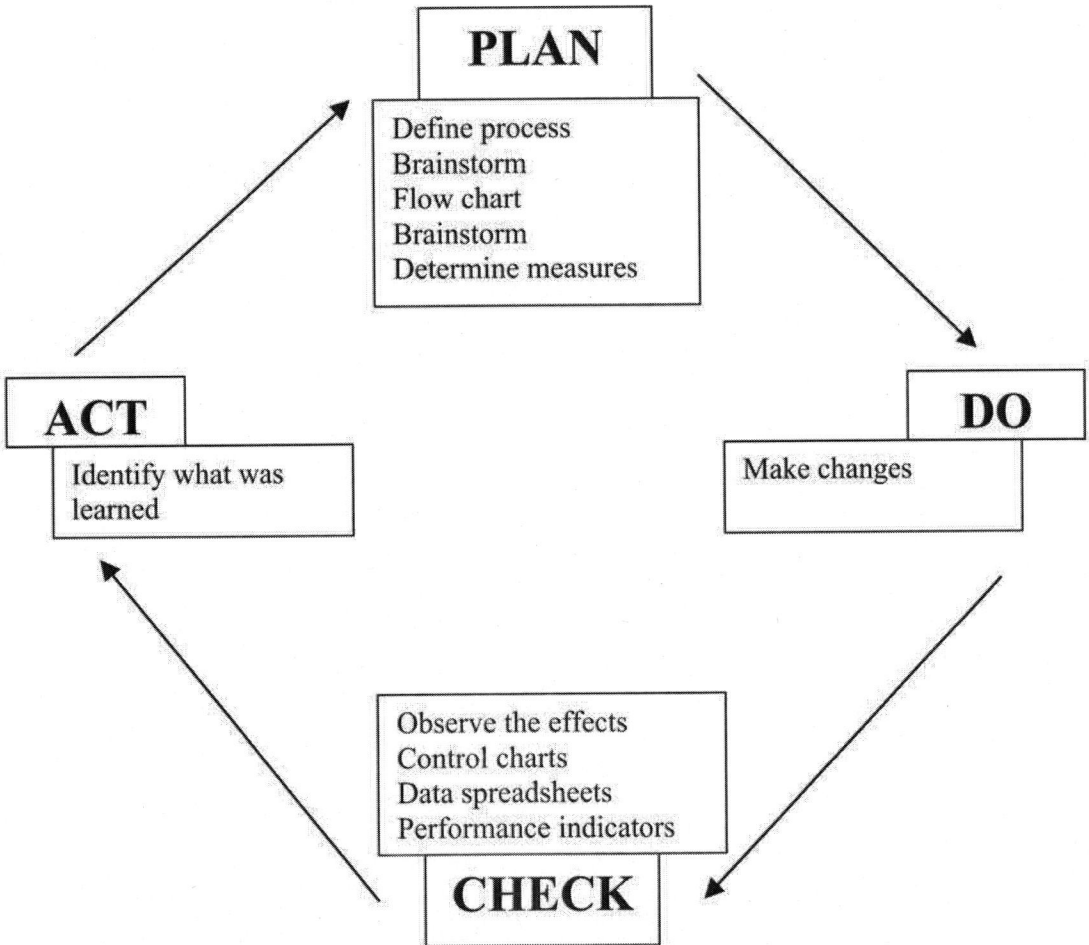

```
                         PLAN
                    ┌─────────────────────┐
                    │ Define process      │
                    │ Brainstorm          │
                    │ Flow chart          │
                    │ Brainstorm          │
                    │ Determine measures  │
                    └─────────────────────┘

   ACT                                           DO
┌──────────────────┐              ┌──────────────────┐
│ Identify what was│              │ Make changes     │
│ learned          │              │                  │
└──────────────────┘              └──────────────────┘

                    ┌─────────────────────┐
                    │ Observe the effects │
                    │ Control charts      │
                    │ Data spreadsheets   │
                    │ Performance indicators│
                    └─────────────────────┘
                        CHECK
```

Source: McLaughlin, C., and A. Kaluzny. 2006. *Continuous quality improvement in health care.* Sudbury, MA: Jones and Bartlett Publishers.

6. Once decision is made, act upon what you decided
7. If you can't reach consensus, take a vote and abide by majority

Quality Improvement

Quality improvement relates to quality of care, quality of life, and safety for residents. It is an ongoing process and is different from **quality assurance**, which looks at the pattern of all actions to ensure that services conform to established technical requirements, regulations, or standards. Quality assurance is an older concept of managing quality. Quality improvement is the desired method in RC/AL facilities for achieving quality outcomes because it is an evolving, dynamic process and is sensitive to the needs of a changing organization.

The quality of care in the RC/AL facility is associated with choice, privacy, independence, security, and autonomy for the resident. Quality of care also assumes that there is quality staff to perform needed services for the residents. The RC/AL facility should measure what quality means to the resident, the resident's family, the staff, regulatory agencies, and stakeholders and allow them to articulate the standards based on their needs. Through a common definition of quality, the facility can embark on a quality improvement program.

Several terms may be used to describe the process of quality improvement. The most common terms are *total quality management* (TQM) or *continuous quality improvement* (CQI). Both TQM and CQI are "structured organizational processes for involving personnel in planning and executing a continuous flow of improvements to provide quality healthcare that meets or exceeds expectations" (McLaughlin and Kaluzny 2006, 3).

Once a definition of quality is established for the facility, the administrator should initiate and establish plans for measuring and improving the quality of the facility. How does an executive define and monitor **quality management** systems? Consider this example. You attend a seminar with two co-workers. Before the first speaker begins, all of you glance around the conference room and begin to notice the cleanliness of the room. One co-worker mentions that the wastebasket near the door is brimming with papers and dirty paper coffee cups. The other wonders what housekeeping uses to keep black heel marks off the floors since the cleaners used by your own housekeeping staff do not seem able to pick them up. The conversation continues in this vein for a few minutes, with all of you noticing and commenting on the general appearance of the conference room—carpets, walls, windows, curtains, and so on. In the end, you will have drafted a list for the housekeeping director to refine and then use in maintaining the cleanliness and appearance of the room (Hughes, Namazi, and Chafetz, in Namazi and Chafetz 2001).

Quality improvement tools can be used to measure quality outcomes, such as flow charts and fishbone diagrams. Flow charts visually represent a workflow process so that it can be evaluated, simplified, or corrected. Fishbone diagrams evaluate all the inputs to a task and identify how each may enhance or impede the process (Namazi and Chafetz 2001). Other instruments can be used such as customer satisfaction surveys. Scorecards for measuring the facility's performance are also popular tools because these items measure performance in areas such as people management, quality of service and care, and financial outcomes (Grant et al. 2006).

The tools for measuring quality in the RC/AL facility are tools that the administrator uses in the management function of controlling and feedback. For example, the PDCA (Plan-Do-Check-Act) Cycle (Figure 5.2) is often used in quality improvement programs. Each of these tools is concerned with measuring the quality of care through establishing a plan, discovering a cause, or developing a pattern. The RC/AL facility administrator should be familiar with each of these tools and assist staff in using them appropriately to improve the quality of the facility.

Leadership and Ethics in the Facility

Ethics is the beliefs or attitudes that make up the moral value of the organization. Ethics represent what should be done but not necessarily what must be done (McConnell 2006). For the RC/AL facility administrator, there is an implicit assumption that he or she will lead according to a code of ethics. No specific code of ethics exists for RC/AL facility administrators. The Code of Ethics for the American College of Health Care Administrators is applicable to RC/AL facility administrators (Appendix 5.A).

Day-to-day ethics with the RC/AL facility is primarily concerned with personal autonomy and end-of-life issues. Ethical behaviors that govern the administrator in these day-to-day issues will reflect his or her personal values and the values of the facility. The ethical principles of beneficence, nonmaleficence, and fidelity influence the administrator's role as the leader of the facility. The principle of beneficence is that what is best for each person's welfare should be done. Beneficence is often referred to as doing what is good for the resident. The ethical principle of nonmaleficence, which means to avoid evil and evil consequences unless there is proportionate reason for risking or permitting such evil, essentially means to do no harm. Fidelity in the RC/AL facility requires the administrator be faithful and keep promises.

Autonomy in the RC/AL facility involves the residents' right to make their own decisions. As residents exercise their independence, the ethics of the facility requires that those wishes be granted as much as possible. The staff and administrator should value, encourage, and affirm the residents' autonomy.

In valuing and affirming the residents' autonomy, the administrator and staff must be prepared to address end-of-life issues. Residents' rights to forgo life-sustaining treatment or to determine the amount of care desired during the final stages of life are influenced by the facility's ethics.

As more RC/AL facilities are introducing hospice into the service options, the need for policies regarding end-of-life issues becomes paramount. At a minimum, information should be provided to the residents regarding the creation and execution of advanced directives and end-of-life preferences. Advanced directives may include a living will and a durable power of attorney for healthcare. Advanced directives ensure that the residents are cared for in the manner in which they desire.

Professional Organizations

RC/AL administrators should be aware of a number of professional organizations that provide membership opportunities and services to their constituency, publish research and reports, and hold annual meetings. These are as follows:

- The Assisted Living Federation of America, a national association dedicated to professionally operated assisted living communities for seniors (http://www.alfa.org).
- The American College of Health Care Administrators, a professional organization dedicated to providing educational opportunities and career development to its long term care administrators (http://www.achca.org).
- The American Association of Homes and Services for the Aging and its members serve two million people every day through mission-driven, not-for-profit organizations dedicated to providing the services people need, when they need them, in the place they call home (http://www.aahsa.org).
- The American Health Care Association, a nonprofit federation of affiliated state health organizations representing more than 10,000 nonprofit and for-profit assisted living, nursing facility, developmentally disabled, and subacute care providers (http://www.ahca.org).
- The National Center for Assisted Living, the assisted living voice of the American Health Care Association, the nation's largest organization representing long term care (http://www.ncal.org).
- The Administration on Aging, which is the federal focal point and advocate agency for older persons and their concerns (http://www.aoa.dhhs.gov).

GLOSSARY

Administrator: A person who has general administrative charge of the day-to-day operations of an assisted living facility. He or she may be the owner or may be hired by the organization. Licensing and/or certification requirements differ from state to state.

Advisory board: This term has various applications. This board is generally made up of a group of members of a community to relate to top management in various advisory capacities as determined by the organization's by-laws.

Articles of Incorporation: Information filed with a state official (usually secretary of state) by persons wishing to form a corporation. Articles of Incorporation give the corporate name and address, names and addresses of corporate officers, and the purpose of the corporation, and other information as required by a particular state.

Authority: The right of power to act, to decide, and to command others.

Board of directors: A group of people who relate to top management of an organization in a governing or advisory capacity as determined by its by-laws. (*See also* **Governing board** and **Advisory board**)

By-laws: The rules that determine the internal management of a board or organization; the official guidelines from which policies and procedures are developed. By-laws are adopted at the time of charter and define the rights and responsibilities of the board and its officers, the membership and its voting privileges.

Communication: The exchange of information from one source to another in such a manner that it is understood by the receiving source.

Consensus building: A conversational style of decision making whereby issues and opinions are discussed across a range of perspectives with the objective of reaching a shared opinion or compromise agreement among a group of participants.

Controlling: The basic management function that involves the measurement of the performance throughout the entire facility to ensure that organizational goals are being achieved and that corrective action is taken if they are not.

Corporation: This term is used to define the form of business that is incorporated under the laws of one of the states. There may be a single stockholder or there may be thousands. A corporation is a separate legal entity from its stockholders and therefore the owners are not personally liable for the debt of the corporation. Most assisted living facilities are operated as a corporation.

Delegation of authority: The process that a manager uses in assigning duties and responsibilities to a subordinate and giving the subordinate the authority necessary to accomplish the assignment.

Directing: The management function when the administrator uses his or her position to point out the direction the company is to go to achieve its goals by use of a variety of leadership roles to include coaching, guiding, training, persuading, challenging, and encouraging the personnel to attain those goals.

Ethics: A system of moral principles, rules, and standards of conduct.

Feedback: The aspects of the communication loop that lets the sender know whether the message was received.

For-profit: An institution, corporation, or other legal entity that is organized for the profit or benefit of its shareholders or other owners.

Goals or objectives: These are the end points that all organizational activities are directed toward. They should be realistic, verifiable, and attainable.

Governance: The people, policies, and processes that provide the framework within which managers make decisions and take actions to optimize outcomes related to their spheres of responsibility.

Governing boards: This term is frequently applied to the governing body. It exercises authority in the governance of the organization. It is responsible for appointing top management, policy making, and ensuring that the policies are administered in a manner and the spirit in which they were written.

Hierarchy of needs: Theory of human motivation developed by Abraham Maslow. One of the most widely accepted and earliest explanations of why people act and react the way they do. According to this theory, each person is always in the state of needing something. Exactly what is needed is dependent on what needs have already been met.

Influencing: Awareness of the lines of authority and the power structure in the organization is an important aspect of understanding the operating culture. Oftentimes, individuals within an organization try to exert influence over others, to persuade them toward (or away from) a course of action.

Job descriptions: Descriptions that define in writing the responsibilities, requirements, functions, duties, location, environment, conditions, and other aspects of jobs.

Laissez-faire: The philosophy of "leave it alone," or nonintervention.

Managing risk: A program of policies and procedures that is established by the administrator as a proactive means of anticipating problems in the facility that could lead to illness, injury, or financial loss.

Management: Is the ability to achieve common goals through the organization and productivity of other people. It involves creating and maintaining an environment in the organization that makes it possible for people to work together to contribute to the accomplishment of the organization's objectives with the least amount of friction possible.

Mission statement: A statement of the purpose of an organization and its reason for existing. It is usually rather brief (less than a page) and does not present detailed information about the day-to-day operations of the organization.

Negotiated risk: A process of negotiating the way that services are going to be provided in dealing with exceptions, unusual circumstances, or problem situations outside the regular practices and service plans.

Not-for-profit: An organization operated solely for social welfare, or for any other purpose except for profit; no part of the organization's income is payable to, or is otherwise available for the personal benefit of, any proprietor or member.

Ombudsman: A person trained to provide advocacy and liaison for elderly residents of healthcare facilities regarding the actions of an administrative nature that affect the resident's health, safety, welfare, or rights. The Ombudsman Program is nationally funded by the Administration on Aging and administered by state agencies.

Organizational chart: A diagrammatic representation of the organization. It displays the lines of formal communication, and authority. It also graphically represents the framework of the organizational structure and the relationships of the different positions and departments to one another.

Organizing: A basic management function through which the formal structure of the organization is established to facilitate the development and allocation of authority and resources throughout the entire organization. It involves the grouping of people and activities, the assigning of roles, and the delegation of authority.

Participative: A management style that encourages managers to share their knowledge and opinions and work together to produce change and organizational results.

Partnership: This term is used to define a business that is owned by two or more persons associated as partners. One or more partners are usually involved in the management of the business. Partners are personally liable for the debt of the business.

Planning: A basic function of management that involves the process of gathering and evaluating information, setting goals, and establishing guidelines that will lead to their accomplishment.

Policies: These are the general statements that guide the thinking and decision making of the assisted living facility staff. Because they are guides for decision making, policies must allow for some discretion to be exercised by the decision maker.

Procedures: These are step-by-step guides to action that establish a required method for handling future activities.

79

Quality assurance: A planned and systematic pattern of all actions necessary to ensure that services conform to established technical requirements or standards.

Quality improvement: A method of evaluating and improving processes of resident care that emphasizes a multidisciplinary approach to problem solving and focuses not on individuals but systems of resident care that might be the cause of variations.

Quality management: A broad term that encompasses both quality assurance and quality improvement, and describes a program of evaluating the quality of care using a variety of methodologies and techniques.

Regulations: Rules by which a statute is specifically implemented on a day-to-day basis by an administrative agency at the federal, state, or local level. A law that has been coded and advertised and is to be monitored by a specific regulatory agency.

Representing: The management function of being the spokesperson for the assisted living organization to residents and their families, government entities, other health-related organizations, and the public.

Rules: These are specific commands that spell out required action or nonaction. They allow no discretion at all.

Shared responsibility: This term means exploring the options available to a resident in a facility and the risks involved with each option when making decisions pertaining to the resident's abilities, preferences, and service needs, thereby enabling the resident and, if applicable, the resident's representative or designee, and the facility to develop a service plan or negotiated risk agreement that best meets the resident's needs and seeks to improve the resident's quality of life.

Short-term or operational planning: This is the process of deliberating and selecting goals for a specified period of time, usually a year. These plans must be coordinated with the facility's strategic plan to ensure continuity of the goals and objectives.

Span of management: A principle of management that states that there is a limited number of people that a manager can effectively supervise.

Staffing: Assigning a person to the execution of the process or an activity.

Strategic planning: The process that an organization uses to reevaluate its mission, identify its long-term and short-term goals, and select its strategies and policies for achieving those goals.

Strategies: These are the general plans of action and deployment of resources that focus on the attainment of the goals of the assisted living facility.

Teams: A team comprises any group of people linked in a common purpose.

Team building: Team building is a planned effort made to improve communications and working relationships by way of any planned and managed change involving a group of people. Team building is most effective when used as a part of a long-range strategy for organizational and personal development.

Vision statement: A statement giving a broad, inspirational image of the future that an organization is aiming to achieve.

PRACTICE QUESTIONS

Read each item carefully, and then select the best response.

1. The resident negotiated risk agreement would *not* include which of the following?
   A. Areas in which the facility assumes liability
   B. The resident's special preferences and needs
   C. The ability of a facility to respond
   D. Evaluation of possible outcomes

   A B C D
   o o o o

2. The ultimate goal of an administrator is to:
   A. establish a high-quality working environment.
   B. maintain sustained profitability.
   C. motivate residents and staff.
   D. achieve organizational effectiveness.

   A B C D
   o o o o

3. What is the purpose of the facility's mission statement?
   A. Convince government to invest in the well-being of the elderly
   B. To list the company's intention and its reason for existing.
   C. Demonstrate desired policies for residents' rights and needs
   D. Influence society to accept and value assisted living

   A B C D
   o o o o

4. An administrator who is a leader is best represented by which of the following terms?
   A. Representing
   B. Organizing
   C. Controlling
   D. Directing

   A B C D
   o o o o

5. The strategic plan for an RC/AL will:
   A. outline goals, objectives, and priorities to achieve the facility's mission.
   B. indicate the facility's lines of communication and authority.
   C. recommend standards and information systems.
   D. focus on staffing and training systems to achieve an effective team.

   A B C D
   o o o o

6. When a group of individuals comes together to accomplish a goal or purpose, this activity is known as what?
   A. Consensus building
   B. Team building
   C. Strategic planning
   D. Union staffing

   A B C D
   o o o o

7. Which of the following is *not* a part of a quality improvement program?
   A. Determining ways of being a spokesperson for the facility
   B. Establishing standards for all aspects of operations
   C. Determining ways to measure performance against standards
   D. Taking corrective action when needed

   A B C D
   ○ ○ ○ ○

8. All of the following are a part of consensus building *except* which one of the following?
   A. Agreement on the objectives for the task or project
   B. Come up with possible resolutions
   C. Not allowing for group compromise
   D. Defining the problem or decision to be reached

   A B C D
   ○ ○ ○ ○

9. What is the purpose of a facility's vision statement?
   A. Convince government to invest in the well-being of the elderly
   B. To list where the company sees itself in the future
   C. Demonstrate desired policies for residents' rights and needs
   D. To describe broad goals for which the company was formed

   A B C D
   ○ ○ ○ ○

10. The primary characteristics of an RC/AL facility *do not* include which of the following?
    A. Privacy
    B. Organizational structure
    C. Social well-being
    D. Independence

    A B C D
    ○ ○ ○ ○

ANSWERS AND EXPLANATIONS

1. **Correct answer = A.** A negotiated risk agreement does not cover areas in which the facility assumes liability.
2. **Correct answer = D.** The primary role of an administrator is to make sure that an organization works effectively to achieve its goals and objectives.
3. **Correct answer = B.** The mission statement is a statement of the purpose of an organizations and its reason for existing. It lists broad goals for which the company was formed.
4. **Correct answer = D.** Directing involves influencing behavior through motivation, communication, leadership, and discipline.
5. **Correct answer = A.** Strategic planning requires the administrator to work with stakeholders to determine the appropriate allocation of resources necessary to achieve the goals and objectives established by the facility's mission statement.
6. **Correct answer = B.** When a team comes together and directs energy toward problem solving, task effectiveness, and accomplishing a goal or purpose, this is known as team building.
7. **Correct answer = A.** A quality improvement program establishes standards, measures performance, and takes corrective action; it has nothing to do with being a spokesperson for the facility.
8. **Correct answer = C.** Consensus building produces a team agreement and must allow for compromise.
9. **Correct answer = B.** A vision statement guides what a company wants to be. It lists where the company sees itself some years from now.
10. **Correct answer = B.** An RC/AL facility's organizational structure is not one of its primary characteristics.

REFERENCES

Borowski, N. 2005. *Organizational Behavior in Health Care*. Sudbury, MA: Jones and Bartlett.

Davis, W., R. Haacker, and J. Townsend. 2002. *The Principles of Health Care Administration*. Bossier City, LA: Professional Printing & Publishing, Inc.

Dunn, R. 2002. *Haimann's Healthcare Management*. 7th ed. Chicago: Health Administration Press.

Francis, D., and D. Young. 1979. *Improving Work Groups: A Practical Manual for Team Building*. San Diego, CA: University Associates.

Grant, Leslie A., Janice Gulsvig, and Jeff Call. 2006. *Measuring Excellence: The New Quality Agenda*. My InnerView. Provider (October), http://www.myinnerview.com/news/2006_Oct_Provider.pdf.

Kelly, D. 2003. *Applying Quality Management in Healthcare: A Process for Improvement*. Chicago: Health Administration Press.

Liebler, J., and C. McConnell. 2004. *Management Principles for Health Professionals*. 4th ed. Sudbury, MA: Jones and Bartlett Publishers.

McConnell, C. 2006. *Umiker's Management Skills for the New Health Care Supervisor*. 4th ed. Sudbury, MA: Jones and Bartlett Publishers.

McLaughlin, C. and A. Kaluzny. 2006. *Continuous Quality Improvement in Health care*. Sudbury, MA: Jones and Bartlett.

Namazi, K.H., and P.K. Chafetz, eds. 2001. *Assisted Living: Current Issues in Facility Management and Resident Care*. Westport, CT: Auburn House.

Northouse, P. 2004. *Leadership: Theory and Practice*. 3rd ed. Thousand Oaks, CA: Sage Publications.

Triton and Patterns Project, Technology Grants. 2000. *Process Guide #2, Building Consensus*. http://projects.edtech.sandi.net/staffdev/tpss99/processguides/consensus.html

Zimmerman, S., P. Sloane, and J. Eckert, eds. 2001. *Assisted Living: Needs, Practices, and Policies in Residential Care for the Elderly*. Baltimore: Johns Hopkins University Press.

AMERICAN COLLEGE OF HEALTH CARE ADMINISTRATORS CODE OF ETHICS

Preamble:

The preservation of the highest standards of integrity and ethical principles is vital to the successful discharge of the professional responsibilities of all long term health care administrators. The American College of Health Care Administrators (ACHCA) has promulgated this Code of Ethics in an effort to stress the fundamental rules considered essential to this basic purpose. It shall be the obligation of members to seek to avoid not only conduct specifically proscribed by the code, but also conduct that is inconsistent with its spirit and purpose. Failure to specify any particular responsibility or practice in this Code of Ethics should not be construed as denial of the existence of other responsibilities or practices. Recognizing that the ultimate responsibility for applying standards and ethics falls upon the individual, the ACHCA establishes the following Code of Ethics to make clear its expectation of the membership.

EXPECTATION I

Individuals shall hold paramount the welfare of persons for whom care is provided.

Prescriptions: The Health Care Administrator shall:

- Strive to provide to all those entrusted to his or her care the highest quality of appropriate services possible in light of resources or other constraints.

- Operate the facility consistent with laws, regulations, and standards of practice recognized in the field of health care administration.
- Consistent with law and professional standards, protect the confidentiality of information regarding individual recipients of care.
- Perform administrative duties with the personal integrity that will earn the confidence, trust, and respect of the general public.
- Take appropriate steps to avoid discrimination on the basis of race, color, sex, religion, age, national origin, handicap, marital status, ancestry, or any other factor that is illegally discriminatory or not related to bona fide requirements of quality care.

Proscription: The Health Care Administrator shall not:

- Disclose professional or personal information regarding recipients of service to unauthorized personnel unless required by law or to protect the public welfare.

EXPECTATION II

Individuals shall maintain high standards of professional competence.

Prescriptions: The Health Care Administrator shall:

84

- Possess and maintain the competencies necessary to effectively perform his or her responsibilities.
- Practice administration in accordance with capabilities and proficiencies and, when appropriate, seek counsel from qualified others.
- Actively strive to enhance knowledge of and expertise in long term care administration through continuing education and professional development.

Proscriptions: The Health Care Administrator shall not:

- Misrepresent qualifications, education, experience, or affiliations.
- Provide services other than those for which he or she is prepared and qualified to perform.

EXPECTATION III

Individuals shall strive, in all matters relating to their professional functions, to maintain a professional posture that places paramount the interests of the facility and its residents.

Prescriptions: The Health Care Administrator shall:

- Avoid partisanship and provide a forum for the fair resolution of any disputes which may arise in service delivery or facility management.
- Disclose to the governing body or other authority as may be appropriate, any actual or potential circumstance concerning him or her that might reasonably be thought to create a conflict of interest or have a substantial adverse impact on the facility or its residents.

Proscription: The Health Care Administrator shall not:

- Participate in activities that reasonably may be thought to create a conflict of interest or have the potential to have a substantial adverse impact on the facility or its residents.

EXPECTATION IV

Individuals shall honor their responsibilities to the public, their profession, and their relationships with colleagues and members of related professions.

Prescriptions: The Health Care Administrator shall:

- Foster increased knowledge within the profession of health care administration and support research efforts toward this end.
- Participate with others in the community to plan for and provide a full range of health care services.
- Share areas of expertise with colleagues, students, and the general public to increase awareness and promote understanding of health care in general and the profession in particular.
- Inform the ACHCA Standards and Ethics Committee of actual or potential violations of this Code of Ethics, and fully cooperate with ACHCA's sanctioned inquiries into matters of professional conduct related to this Code of Ethics.

Proscription: The Health Care Administrator shall not:

- Defend, support, or ignore unethical conduct perpetrated by colleagues, peers or students.

Source: American College of Healthcare Administrators, http://www.achca.org.

LISA J. SCHAAF YEHL, MHSA, LHNA, has a bachelor of science in business administration from Central Michigan University with a minor in public health administration and a master of health services administration from Ohio University. She worked as an assistant administrator for Hickory Creek Nursing Center; served as an interim administrator at Eagle Creek Nursing Center in West Union, Ohio. Licensed nursing home administrator (LNHA) 1991–2005. Ohio University interim instructor 2002–2005; full-time instructor 2005–present; program coordinator for long term healthcare administration program.

For 25 years DELVIN ZOOK, RC/AL administrator and CEO, has been the director of Rock of Ages Mennonite Home (RCF), Valley View Retirement Village, and an in-home care agency. Delvin designed and developed the Valley View Retirement Village, including in-home services. He served as president (2000–2002) on the board of directors for the Oregon Alliance of Senior and Health Services. He serves on the House of Delegates for the American Association of Homes and Services for the Aging. He has served on various committees for the state of Oregon, including rewriting RC/AL rules and regulations. One of the original item writers for NAB's RC/AL administrator exam, Delvin continues to serve on various NAB committees.

CHAPTER 6

PHYSICAL ENVIRONMENT MANAGEMENT

Lisa J. Schaaf Yehl, MHSA, LNHA
Delvin Zook

Introduction

The physical environment of the residential care/assisted living (RC/AL) facility is key to the reception it receives from its community, its staff, and its residents. The decoration of the facility not only affects "curbside appeal" for those who visit but also affects the ongoing satisfaction of the residents who have chosen to reside there. It also becomes important that the environment be well maintained, not only for safety reasons but for the continued success of the facility. Local, state, and federal laws establish requirements that affect the residence and its environment. These laws also direct program requirements after the facility has been opened.

RC/AL residences must also comply with the same regulations relating to resident and employee safety (e.g., the Occupational Safety and Health Act, **Life Safety Code**) and employee rights (e.g., requirements of the **Equal Employment Opportunity Commission**, **Family Medical Leave Act**) that other provider organizations do (Pratt 2003).

The physical environment of an RC/AL facility was one of the driving factors when developing a new philosophy of care for frail and elderly persons. As early as the 1980s, certain states took lead roles in a new concept and design that would provide housing and services outside of the traditional way of caring for elderly people. Other states soon followed, and today almost every state has some type of community-based care settings where frail and elderly people are cared for outside of nursing home settings. At this time, there is minimal federal regulation of RC/AL facilities, and so each state has facilities designed differently. The design may look different from state to state, but the ultimate goal is to create a homelike setting for frail and elderly persons.

Models of RC/AL Care and the Physical Environment

How can a safe and secure environment be provided for the elderly in a "homelike" setting and yet meet all the local, state, and federal guidelines and regulations? The administrator must know the difference between the **social model** and **medical model of care** for RC/AL facilities. The goal of the social model is to provide holistic care by meeting all needs of a resident, including healthcare, at the level the facility provides. The administrator must take precautions dealing with the concept of aging in place. Each resident will become more frail and have added mobility and health issues. The administrator must have policies in place that deal with such issues. Some facility policies require a move if the level of care necessary surpasses a level that can be provided safely by the facility. Some residents may have additional nursing care needs that become a challenge to provide in a homelike environment.

Strong, "hidden" nursing support must be in place and should be supported by written facility policy.

The medical model, such as that implemented in a nursing facility or hospital setting, has very defined goals to make people well or at least to provide care; the main focus is on the medical needs of the person. The restructuring of long term care in recent years, especially in community-based systems such as RC/AL residences, focuses more on the social needs and individual choices of the resident. Sometimes the choices residents make conflict with their medical needs. For example, a diabetic elderly person needs to live in a safe environment where staff are available to assist with health issues when necessary rather than living in the person's own home with the simple instruction not to eat candy because it will affect the diabetes.

The medical model emphasizes the appropriate steps to take to make and keep a person healthy. The social model places more emphasis on a personal choice of individuals rather than the medical consequences of those choices. This is why a strong, hidden nursing support system is so important and an obligation of the facility to provide holistic care in the RC/AL system. If at any time a resident's medical needs become unstable or unpredictable, generally most RC/AL facilities are not equipped to deliver such care (Allen 2004).

State and Local Regulations and the RC/AL Facility

In any community, in which you desire to build an RC/AL, many laws and rules exist to guide the owner and/or limit the freedom with which the facility is constructed. Local **zoning laws** specify which properties are for commercial buildings as opposed to residential homes. The local city council, which serves as a gatekeeper for the community, might need to approve the proposed RC/AL facility architectural drawings and plans before construction can begin. Buildings must

also be constructed of acceptable materials to maintain the safety of occupants, the surrounding neighborhood, and the rights of way and roads used for local traffic. Local **building codes** may also require permits for construction so that there is an oversight process in place to approve the construction of the facility at each phase.

Some states may require a certificate of need before allowing additional beds or a new RC/AL facility to be constructed. This requirement is similar to the one for licensed nursing facilities in states such as New Jersey. The developer must prove there is a need for the facility in the community by a process governed by the state. This requirement protects communities from overdeveloping RC/AL facilities, which can cause high vacancy rates and create a strain on already-existing facilities and the system. Some states, such as Oregon, may even place a moratorium on construction of new facilities for a period of time for the same purpose. Most states, however, do not have regulations requiring a certificate of need for RC/AL facilities.

Regulation is for the safety and protection of the consumer, but can create other challenges for the administrator. Administrators must ensure the facility complies with federal laws such as the **Americans with Disabilities Act (ADA)**, the Occupational Health and Safety Act (OSHA), **National Fire Protection Association**/Life Safety Code (NFPA), and others. However, meeting all of the regulations, such as the display of all required informational signs and posters, can detract from the homelike atmosphere the RC/AL facility works to attain. Each facility should have a designated bulletin board or other means to meet regulation posting requirements that does not distract from the homelike setting.

Residents and community members will either perceive the RC/AL facility as one with that homelike feel or one that is institutionalized. To minimize the institutional feel, the administrator must make decisions that affect the living environment. In more recent years, vendors of furniture and other home necessities have developed a large selection of commercial-grade furniture that is meant to serve the elderly population and yet does not detract from the homelike setting. The administrator must follow standards required by the National Fire Protection Association/ Life Safety Code (NFPA) when choosing fire-retardant materials for draperies, furniture, mattresses, and other fittings. The RC/AL administrator must also maintain documentation verifying that these requirements have been met in the facility's purchases. The state fire marshal can provide more information on these issues.

The administrator can affect the home environment by introducing room designs and décor that either add to or detract from the desired results. For example, the nurses' station can diminish the home environment if not properly designed or placed within the facility. As a resolution, the administrator might consider a design in which the nurses' station is hidden by a private dining room look, with residential kitchen cabinets designed for pullout computer stations. Such a design would provide the needed space for a strong nursing program, which includes staff conferencing, yet would not distract from the home feel. If new RC/AL facility construction is planned, administrators must carefully consider which architect is hired for the design of the new building to ensure an architect that is knowledgeable about and understands the concept and philosophy of assisted living is hired.

Ongoing Evaluation of the RC/AL Environment

The administrator must commit to ongoing evaluation of both the facility environment and services. Staff in-service training programs on the RC/AL philosophy and standards must be in place. New employees coming from nursing home settings may not understand the philosophy of assisted living. In addition, staff turnover problems may

reduce the time invested in employee orientation. Not providing proper staff orientation and training can inadvertently affect the residents' living environment and cost the administrator more time and money to recapture the original living environment.

Implementation of Policies, Conflict Resolution, and Environmental Impact

The RC/AL administrator is a role model to the staff and should ensure that the policies and procedures of the organization are implemented properly. This translates into how residents, as well as family members, vendors, and all other stakeholders of the facility, are treated by the staff and administrator. Occasionally, conflicts may arise with staff and residents, and if the administrator handles the problems appropriately, it can strengthen the work environment in the RC/AL. In the event a policy or procedure is no longer effective, a **continuous quality improvement (CQI)** committee should be formed by the administrator to address the issue. This committee can recommend necessary changes.

The administrator is also responsible for prioritizing the use of organizational resources in accordance with the goals established for the RC/AL. These decisions affect daily operations, financial solvency, quality of care provided to the residents, and future decisions.

Regulatory Compliance for RC/AL Facilities

RC/AL facilities must comply with regulations that govern the operation of all businesses in the long term care field. The administrator must be knowledgeable of the legal aspects of operation and ensure that they are addressed appropriately in the daily organizational practices. The following are key regulations.

The Fair Housing Amendments Act

The Fair Housing Amendments Act (FHAA) of 1988 allows for the exemption of people with select health problems from participating in the healthcare benefits of the community, but admission cannot be denied unless these people have a contagious disease that can pose a threat to others. Renters can be allowed to modify their own living units at their own expense to accommodate special needs. However, operators can require tenants to restore their units to their original condition upon the termination of their residency, and can require the establishment of an escrow account to provide for such restoration. The FHAA also states that covered facilities cannot deny or limit services nor can their management assign residents to a special floor or section (Pearce 1998).

Americans with Disabilities Act

The purpose of the Americans with Disabilities Act (ADA) in regard to the physical environment of an RC/AL facility is to set guidelines for providing accessibility for individuals with disabilities. These guidelines must be applied during the design, construction, and alteration of facilities (Allen 2004). ADA guidelines were developed to meet the "public" need to have access to public areas. ADA does not affect the construction of private homes, but when the public is involved, where employees, visitors, and residents must access facilities, construction and renovations must meet ADA guidelines.

Because ADA affects residents and employees of RC/AL facilities, consideration should be given to meet the requirements and yet not detract from the desired homelike environment. For example, an RC/AL facility can make the "reasonable accommodation" of providing wheelchair access for residents with disabilities without negatively affecting the cosmetics of the facility environment.

Occupational Safety and Health Act

The Occupational Safety and Health Act (OSHA) requires the implementation of specific programs to protect employees and residents from hazards and unsafe working conditions. OSHA reporting requirements are generally applicable to any employer with 11 or more employees. Areas to be addressed include the following:

1. *Posting the OSHA notice* in a prominent location. This notice informs workers of their rights under the law. All employers regardless of size must display this poster. Hazard communication standards and imminent danger notices must also be included with the posting.
2. *Appropriate safety equipment* such as goggles, eye wash stations and first aid kits, and properly rated ladders and tools must be made available to ensure worker safety and rapid responses to emergencies as they arise.
3. *A comprehensive hazard communication program* must be established so that all staff, residents, and visitors are aware of and understand how to access needed information. Employees of an RC/AL residence have a **right to know** what chemicals they may be using in their day-to-day work, what the potential hazards of such chemicals may be, and how to protect themselves from danger. The administrator must ensure that all employees are provided education and training about the use of protective equipment, and this protective equipment, such as rubber gowns, gloves, and goggles for use in laundry and containers for proper disposal of hazardous materials, must be made available in each department. Each department must have proper equipment that correlates with the jobs performed by employees in that department, and the equipment should be readily accessible.

The facility must also have **Material Safety Data Sheets (MSDSs)** available in each department. An inventory of all products used by the employees that could present a hazard, such as soaps, cleaners, and sprays, must have a corresponding MSDS. No product that is purchased is to be put into use until the MSDS is obtained from the manufacturer. Each department must have a clearly labeled red notebook or binder in which the MSDS are kept along with an alphabetical listing in front of all MSDSs contained in the binder. This makes for ease of access to the appropriate MSDS in case of an emergency. A complete set of MSDS for the entire facility must be kept in a central location, in case no one is in the corresponding department at the time the emergency occurs. This ensures the MSDS can be faxed to the emergency department for use by the attending physician in case of an emergency. MSDSs for products no longer in use in the RC/AL facility must be maintained in a separate binder and maintained for a period of 30 years. Corresponding documentation proving education of all staff must also be maintained in the event any issues arise in the future.

4. A *"lock out tag out" requirement* for any electrical work to ensure the safety of staff. A complete inventory of all equipment must be performed by the administrator or his or her designee who possesses the necessary skills to do so safely. Documentation is necessary showing the power source for each piece of equipment, the department in which the equipment is located, the voltage of electrical power, the method in which the equipment is disconnected from its power source, and those individuals who will be affected when the equipment is in need of repair. The documentation must also include who will notify those individuals affected by the equipment slated for repair, as well as documentation of the notification of those individuals affected by repair of the equipment.

Once repairs to the equipment have been completed, only the individual who possesses the necessary skills may remove the lock and/or tag from the equipment and deem it ready for use. All individuals who have been affected by the repair of the equipment must be notified that repairs have been completed and that equipment is now ready for use. This must also be documented by date and time, and individuals notified and maintained in the permanent records of the LockOut/TagOut Program.

5. *A proactive safety program* that includes a regular program of hazard identification (such as safety rounds), documentation of all significant incidents, and employee safety training.

OSHA requires that employee work-related injury and illnesses be documented on an OSHA 300 Log and OSHA 301 Log, posted annually (February 1st–March 1st) for employee review and retained for five years. A separate log must be maintained for needlestick injuries. OSHA requires that when a needlestick injury occurs, if the investigation reveals that nursing staff did not follow the RC/AL safety policy relating to safe use of needles, the staff member must be disciplined and records maintained. The employee must then be educated about the ramifications of the needlestick, testing services must be offered, and confidential documentation of the test results must be retained in the employee's file. Sharps containers must also be maintained in all areas in which needle usage is more likely to occur along with a policy relating to when these dispensers must be emptied and maintained.

The RC/AL administrator is responsible for ensuring that OSHA regulations are followed and that documentation regarding training in these programs is also maintained. OSHA requires that

91

any employee who states he or she has experienced an "alleged work-related injury" follow the steps of a reporting system established by the RC/AL facility, and usually must report the incident immediately to their supervisor or within a 24-hour period. An accident/incident report must be completed by the employee and an investigation of the incident/accident must be specified by the established program. An employee must report any work-related fatality or in-patient hospitalization of three or more employees within 8 hours to the OSHA area office.

6. *An infection control program* must be established and monitored by the RC/AL administrator. The purpose and intent of this program are to protect staff and residents and to prevent the spread and/or transmission of communicable diseases. Each facility should address key infection control issues such as follows:

a. Methods for identifying, documenting, and investigating infectious diseases

b. Procedures to reduce the risk and prevent the spread of infectious diseases

c. Staff training on issues such as universal precautions, handwashing techniques, linen handling, hazardous waste disposal, proper use of protective equipment, and other means of controlling infections

d. Proper use of disinfectants and germicides to ensure effectiveness

e. Procedures for employee health including evaluations and work restrictions for any employee with communicable diseases or conditions such as flu virus, etc.

f. Designating an area in which sharps containers are kept, locked and safe from residents and staff until pickup of waste has occurred. The facility should initiate contract services with a waste disposal company for pickup and disposal of sharps containers as well as leaving a manifest. The manifest indicates the number of containers picked up, the weight of the containers picked up, and the date and time the containers were picked up. (Small centers could have other ways of disposal such as by dropping off containers at locations for hazardous waste; but small facilities *must* have a plan and policy in place that never allows sharps to be discarded with a regular disposal system.) Should the facility waste exceed a certain weight of sharps containers and/or hazardous materials (bloody bandages, etc.), then the RC/AL facility must register as a large generator of hazardous materials.

Responsibility for implementation, training, monitoring and reporting of this program falls to the nursing supervisor or director of nursing services for a large RC/AL facility. Specifics of the program must be in writing, and training for the infection control program is initiated on hire of new employees as well as periodically and annually for all staff. Data collected as an integral part of this program should be monitored and trends that require intervention noted.

7. *Medical device reporting* is also required by OSHA with the oversight of this requirement by the **Food and Drug Administration**. This requirement is intended to provide notification to the manufacturer as well as a reporting requirement when equipment does not function or perform in the manner specified by the manufacturer, when used per the manufacturer's instruction. For example, a shower chair used within the weight limits specified by the manufacturer breaks during use. If breakage causes injury to the resident, reporting must occur. This important requirement must be monitored by the administrator.

The Life Safety Code and the National Fire Protection Association

The National Fire Protection Association (NFPA) is a nonprofit voluntary membership organization whose sole objective is the reduction of fire, waste of lives, and property. NFPA prepares standards and codes for various types of organizations and facilities. The NFPA is not an enforcement body, but other organizations often adopt and enforce its standards. For long term care facilities, the single most important NFPA standard is the 2000 version of the Life Safety Code NFPA No. 101. These standards were revised by the Technical Committee on Board and Care Facilities to cover **assisted living facilities (ALFs)** (Wolf 2002). The standards mandate that every administration have written copies of a fire plan, practice regular fire drills for each shift, use smoke detectors and sprinklers, and provide training in life safety procedures and devices. Additional regulations cover use of furnishings and draperies that are not combustible and that do not interfere with smoke detectors and sprinklers, as well as construction requirements such as placement and size of doors, ramps and exits, emergency power, and lighting (Allen 2004).

Mechanical, Electrical, Plumbing, and Energy Conservation Standards

Similar to the National Fire Protection Agency (NFPA) there are national organizations that make huge contributions toward safety and uniformity concerning plumbing and electrical systems. Safety and acceptable standards are always concerns for consumers.

The International Association of Plumbing and Mechanical Organization (IAPMO) has been in existence since 1945 aggressively promoting uniform plumbing standards to best serve hundreds of communities and jurisdictions. Because each state and local governments choose to adopt such standards, each residential care/assisted living facility must work with local state and/or county jurisdiction to determine the plumbing guidelines.

Other requirements affect the plumbing systems such as water temperatures supplied for resident access. Other guidelines regulate water temperature used for laundry and dishwashing. Every administrator must know what is required in each area and department.

The electricity that flows through the building powers most systems, from heating, lighting, to mechanical. The electrical system can be very dangerous. The National Electrical Code (NEC) is a national organization that promotes standards that state and local jurisdictions adopt. Electrical standards are fairly uniform, but each residential care/ assisted living facility must check local codes when constructing or renovating buildings.

Poor electrical wiring in walls and attics is a huge fire hazard, and so systems need to be continually checked for deficiencies. The use of electrical cords also can be a major hazard if not maintained properly. Each facility must check local codes as to the use of extension cords.

Conserving energy, whether electricity, gas, or other forms, should be addressed, and programs to conserve should be developed. Having a preventative maintenance program to maintain weather stripping around windows and doors is important. Having adequate insulation for the building not only addresses energy cost savings, but will help make systems operate better and allow residents to be more comfortable.

Safety and Security Requirements and Procedures

The safety and security of the RC/AL resident is ultimately the responsibility of the administrator. The administrator is responsible for ensuring that staff are adequately trained on how to maintain the safety and security of the residents and to whom safety and security issues are reported. This can be accomplished in simple ways such as follows:

1. Include information in the new employee orientation program along

with periodic updates during in-service education programs. These programs should include specialized training in how to care for residents with special needs such as Alzheimer's and related dementias. This will ensure that all employees are instructed in the same manner. Updates may need to be made to the program from time to time.

2. Make sure that employees are trained on what to do and who to notify if a resident is not accounted for during routine rounds and or during a head count. This is commonly known as an *elopement protocol*. An effective elopement protocol includes the following important components: facility policy that defines elopement and all of the program's components, individual staff responsibilities, a facility diagram that depicts all areas in which a resident could become lost and that must be searched, a notebook with pictures and identifying characteristics of the residents who are at risk for elopement (as assessed on move-in) that is updated regularly by the admissions director or designee, and a search kit that contains tools needed in the event a resident has become lost (search cards prepared for each designated search area, flashlights, new batteries, walkie-talkies, rain parkas, diagram depicting all identified areas of the facility that must be searched as well as the protocol that specifically designates which staff member is responsible for all search steps at the time the search protocol is initiated). All components of the program will ensure that staff awareness of safety and security of residents is continuous.

3. A maintenance repair order form should be readily available for use by staff, visitors, or family members. Items that do not pose an immediate danger are written down, including location of repair, nature of repair, date repair is requested, as well as the signature of the individual requesting the repair, and the maintenance request is placed in a central mailbox or designated area known by all staff. Safety issues that an employee believes is an "immediate or imminent danger" to the safety and security of residents must be addressed right away, and staff must be trained in how to do so and to whom the immediate or imminent danger must be reported once it has been identified. Documentation must then be prepared and maintained denoting the immediate danger of the needed repair, who identified the needed repair, and who completed the repair immediately.

Hazardous areas such as boiler rooms, utility rooms, and soiled laundry rooms, must be kept locked and secured when not in use to ensure residents do not enter these rooms and become endangered.

Security Programs

The RC/AL facility must be secure at night. Protocols must be in place concerning, for example, which door to leave open for entrance to the RC/AL facility, at what hour doors will be locked (a fire exit door cannot be locked), how emergency vehicles gain entrance after dark, visitation hours (if those have been established), deliveries that may or may not be accepted after dark, and so forth. An important component of security is exterior lighting as well as employee parking and visitor parking. Employees must understand what practices are acceptable and must be encouraged to ensure the security of the RC/AL facility at all hours of the day or night.

Security is a broad term referring to measures taken to ensure protection and safety of residents, staff, visitors, and the physical plant. Security means more than physical protection and, therefore, includes a variety of other protective measures. Location of the facility is an important factor to consider in security planning. Some of the measures to take for protection of residents are the following:

1. Make sure the building and parking areas of the facility are well lit.
2. Make sure that monitoring devices are used to protect wandering residents. The courts have held that if a facility has a monitoring device and intentionally turns it off for staff convenience, liability may be attributed to the facility.
3. The use of security guards often are needed in high-crime areas, especially during the evening hours. Security guards should make regular rounds inside and outside the building. A close relationship with local law enforcement agencies is important.
4. Local law enforcement should be advised as to the security needs of the facility. A routine inspection by local police, particularly during the night shift, is encouraged.
5. Entrances to the facility should all be locked from the outside.
6. Potential hazards on the facility grounds need to be identified and dealt with when possible. (Buttaro 2002)

Environmental safety also applies to all facility personnel, residents, and visitors. Safety is especially significant in a facility, considering the vulnerability of the residents who are unable to care for themselves during emergency situations (fire, disaster, evacuation). Ordinarily, residents with diminished sensory abilities will require more light, more audible speaking and alarms, and simple traffic patterns with visual and memory aids. Special consideration is needed for people with physically disabilities. The entire staff needs to be aware of these aspects of aging and their ramifications. Guidelines for special consideration for accident prevention in the safety program include the following:

1. An in-service training program should be made available to all personnel using heavy equipment and/or special chemicals.
2. The use of wax on corridors and other floors should be discouraged. Throw rugs and stair treads must be secure.
3. Floors should be kept in smooth and unpitted condition.
4. All corridors and exits should be free from excess beds, bedside tables, wheelchairs, magazine racks, and the like.
5. Corridors, stairways, and resident areas must be well lit.
6. Special attention should be paid to uncovered radiators or steam pipes in resident rooms or corridors.
7. Any frayed or defective wiring in resident rooms and other areas must be taken care of immediately.
8. Grab bars around baths and toilet fixtures must be checked periodically to see that they are secure.
9. Fire extinguishers must be serviced a minimum of once a year to ensure proper functioning and refilling. The date of inspection and the signature of the inspector must be recorded, usually on a tag attached to each extinguisher.
10. The thermostatic control on main hot water heaters and tanks must be checked.
11. All food must be kept under cover and all refuse containers covered.
12. An evacuation and safety plan must be available and distributed to all personnel. This plan should be tested a minimum of four times a year per shift or according to state law. The usual practice is to test monthly, rotating tests to the three shifts, amounting to each shift tested quarterly. (Buttaro 2002)

Security risks in an organization may pose a safety threat to residents. Theft from residents by a staff member may be a concern, including theft of drugs. Abuse/neglect cases may occur at times and should always be taken seriously when reported. Checks and balances, including policies on how to deal with such incidents, need to be in place so that such incidents are detected as soon as possible. Reporting steps must be very specific so that staff are well aware of what their responsibilities are and the timelines within which they are responsible for such reporting. Obtaining a criminal history report, through fingerprint checks with the state Bureau of Criminal Investigations, will help decrease the incidence of hiring individuals with a history of such behaviors.

It is recommended that the following policies for accident prevention for residents be implemented:

1. Medications are to be kept under lock and key at all times; narcotics under double lock. Discontinue the use of medicine bottles with smudged labels. Discard all medicines with expired prescription dates.

2. When administering medications, the nurse or nurse delegate must not place them at bedside and leave the room. Medicine labels should be checked three times (i.e., before pouring, while pouring, and before returning to the shelf) before the medication is given to the resident.

3. The names of residents with known allergies must be noted in a conspicuous place both at the nurses' station and on the outside of the resident's chart.

4. Chronic diseases (such as diabetes or arteriosclerosis) requiring a nurse's attention should be noted on the outside of the particular resident's chart.

5. Encourage the use of high-low beds in the facility. (Buttaro 1999)

Disaster and Emergency Preparedness and Recovery

It is of critical importance to have an effective disaster and emergency preparedness program in place. The **disaster preparedness** program addresses what to do in the event of a disaster (floods, hurricanes, prolonged loss of power or heat, tornadoes, fire, bioterrorism, bomb threats, etc.) to ensure the safety of both staff and residents.

Important components of such a program include the following:

1. Transfer agreements (locations, such as hospitals, nursing homes, churches, other RC/AL facilities, etc. who have agreed to accept your residents in the event of an evacuation) that are updated on an annual basis

2. Emergency preparedness training for all staff during new employee orientation and annually during in-service education (the frequency of training may be dependent on the size and location of the RC/AL facility)

3. Policies addressing what staff should do in the event of each type of disaster (who is to be notified, who is responsible for coordinating transfer of residents and their medical records, what each department is to do and what their functions are to be, notification of owner, administrator, family members, medical director, and/or corporate staff, etc.)

4. Transport agreements (developed with transportation agencies that have agreed to transport your residents from your facility to other locations in the event of disaster)

5. Discussion with area facilities and rescue agencies that may be responsible for disaster preparedness of the community in which you are located, for effective planning on a larger scale

6. An individual designated to serve as media spokesperson during and after the disaster

Once a disaster has occurred in your area, the building may require inspection by local regulatory agencies to ensure that it is safe for the return of your residents. Needed repairs and modifications that are required along with follow-up inspection must be completed prior to returning residents to the RC/AL. When approval for occupancy of the building has been granted, documents reflecting this approval must be maintained by both the administrator and maintenance supervisor. Residents and their family members must be contacted, and the return of the residents to the RC/AL facility must be arranged and completed through the transportation arrangements made by the administrator, per transfer agreements developed by the administrator.

Other emergency preparedness agreements for which the administrator is responsible pertain to water, medications, sprinkler system, and any other vital services as designated by the administrator, owners, or board of directors. The administrator is responsible for ensuring that water is available to all residents, staff, and visitors in the event the water supply has been turned off or interrupted. This means that a water agreement must be established with a local vendor who is able to meet the water demands of the RC/AL facility, on an emergency basis, and who will respond to your need for water in a timely basis. Spare water must also be maintained and dated for emergencies.

The administrator, along with the dietary department, is responsible for ensuring that the RC/AL facility has three days worth of spare food along with seven days supply of dry goods that can be used to serve meals in the event of a disaster. These foodstuffs must also be rotated through and maintained according to date of expiration.

A major concern for any administrator should be medication delivery in the event of a disaster. A contractual agreement between a pharmacy and the RC/AL facility must include disaster planning. A system to deliver needed medications to residents is as important during a disaster as it is when systems are under normal operations. The administrator can identify other pharmacies in the local area and include them in a plan to help if the delivery system is interrupted. Having a pre-planned medication delivery system in place will help the facility meet the needs of residents.

The administrator of the RC/AL should also establish a contract for the regular maintenance and emergency repair of the automatic sprinkler system. Regulations typically require that inspections of the system occur at least quarterly, and documentation of inspections must be maintained by the RC/AL administrator. In the event the facility finds its sprinkler system is down for a period of time, an alternate fire watch plan must be implemented. This protocol is very specific and requires that rounds be made of every area of the RC/AL facility every 15 minutes for visual inspection and documentation of the time and by whom the inspection was made, until the sprinkler system is operational. When the sprinkler system is operational, a report must be made and documentation of such notification must be maintained by the RC/AL administrator. The administrator should also notify the facility owner(s) in the event the sprinkler system is down and nonfunctional.

Grounds Maintenance

It is extremely important to maintain the exterior of the RC/AL residence. It is the first impression people have of the RC/AL facility and shows the public your attention to detail. Grounds maintenance encompasses the entire property on which the RC/AL facility is situated. An individual must be designated to be responsible for regularly scheduled tasks, such as lawn mowing, trimming, edging, removal of trash, watering of flowerbeds, exterior paint touchups, and other tasks as are necessary. Other tasks must also be monitored, for example, holes in the driveway and parking lot that must be filled and/or patched, removal of trees or bushes, cleaning of windows, repair of exterior features (roof, gutters, downspouts, hillsides prone to mudslides, etc.), and snow removal and salting of walkways in winter. Depending on the size of the RC/AL facility, grounds maintenance may require the administrator to hire a full-time groundskeeper as well as part-time seasonal help.

It is the responsibility of the administrator to make outdoor rounds with the maintenance supervisor to audit and make suggestions for needed improvements. Any equipment required to maintain the grounds must be planned for in advance so that financial allowances can be made for procurement.

Preventive and Routine Maintenance Plans and Procedures

It is very important to develop and implement a preventive maintenance program (PMP). A PMP helps prolong the life of equipment purchased and ensures its proper functioning. A PMP includes a facility policy that defines the PMP, the types of **preventive maintenance** to be performed on equipment, and the frequency with which preventive maintenance is completed for each piece of equipment. These documents must be maintained by the maintenance supervisor and periodically reviewed by the administrator. The purpose of this review is to help identify which pieces of equipment may need to be repaired or replaced and which equipment is still under warranty.

Examples of a preventive maintenance activity logged into a PMP log might be as follows:

Date	Equipment	Task	Initials
1/20	Weight Scale	Calibration completed weekly	D. W.

The initials of the maintenance supervisor, as well as the date the weight scale is calibrated, is logged and maintained in the PMP log.

This information is also useful during a regulatory inspection to show that regular preventive maintenance is completed on every piece of equipment. In the event that preventive maintenance of particular pieces of equipment can only be done by the manufacturer, documentation of the preventive maintenance must be maintained in the PMP log.

Routine maintenance plans and procedures should also be in place so that prompt and complete repair of facility and/or equipment is completed by the appropriate individuals in a timely manner. An emergency phone log of all repair technicians must be maintained by maintenance staff and a copy should be provided to the general staff so that a qualified maintenance person can be reached when needed.

The administrator is key to the purchase of materials and equipment. The administrator must ensure that all items purchased are appropriate, safe for use with the resident population, and maintained according to the manufacturer's specifications.

Maintenance repair forms that have been completed and a record of repairs completed must be maintained by the maintenance supervisor or the administrator. A monthly safety committee meeting should be held in which the repairs are reviewed. Repairs that are unusual or that indicate a trend must be addressed by the safety committee. An employee incentive program to reward the employee(s) who notices a repair that would have had dire consequences had it not been addressed should be an established program.

Sanitation and Pest Control

Maintaining the sanitation of the RC/AL as well as ensuring pest control is routinely done are very important. The sanitation of the RC/AL refers to cleanliness and is important in several areas: hallways, kitchen, resident rooms, dining rooms, activity rooms, central living areas, external drives, external walkways, and parking areas. Floors, baseboards, and walls in all such areas must be maintained.

It is the responsibility of the administrator to make daily rounds of the RC/AL facility to check that all areas are clean and are being maintained in the proper manner. Taking this responsibility seriously can prevent many problems for the administrator and allows residents to have a much higher quality of life.

It is also the responsibility of the administrator to initiate contractual agreements with vendors to provide pest control services. The contracts should stipulate the size of the RC/AL facility, the services agreed upon, the frequency of expected pest control visits, emergency services available during off hours, and the fee to be charged for services rendered. This agreement should be revisited at least annually to ensure that services are being provided in the expected manner.

The insurance carrier for the RC/AL facility may also require monthly reporting by the administrator for liability coverage. For example, the administrator may be required to provide information about employee turnover, whether the RC/AL facility had any elopements, abuse/neglect investigations, and any fires or other event that could result in litigation. The insurance carrier may also request review of facility in-service education records to ensure staff are being properly trained in their individual departmental functions (nursing assistants are trained on proper lifting techniques, dietary staff know how to turn off the oven in the event of a fire, staff know where fire extinguishers are located etc.). The administrator must also ensure that the facility is appropriately insured for unexpected events.

GLOSSARY

American with Disabilities Act (ADA): Federal law that gives individuals with disabilities opportunity for employment. It requires employers to make reasonable accommodations for persons with disabilities to be employed.

Assisted living facilities (ALFs): A program approach within a prescribed physical structure on a 24-hour basis. Provides and/ or coordinates a range of supportive personal services and may provide various levels of health services.

Building codes: Codes set forth by various local, state, and federal agencies requiring various degrees of application; processes and guidelines to be followed when building or renovating a building.

Centers for Medicare and Medicaid Services (CMS): A federal agency that regulates federal monies that are available for services to individuals who qualify for Medicare and Medicaid. This federal agency prescribes guidelines for state agencies that regulate licensed care facilities.

Continuous quality improvement (CQI): A system put in place that uses various tools such as resident satisfaction surveys and other measures that allow an organization to improve the quality of services based on past performance and future goals.

Disaster preparedness: Preparation and training of staff and residents in the event of an unexpected event of a great magnitude that affects operation of the healthcare facility and ensures the safety of everyone during this event. Disasters include tornadoes, hurricanes, bomb threats, floods, chemical spills (both internal and external), explosions, fires, and electrical outages.

Employee right to know: An integral component of OSHA guidelines that stipulates that employees must be made aware of chemicals they work with in the performance of their job, where the Material Safety Data Sheets are located so that they can read about the chemicals with which they work, and what the hazards of working with those substances may be.

Equal Employment Opportunity Commission: A federal agency that sets guidelines to ensure equal opportunity for employment based on a person's ability to perform the job and does not allow an employer to discriminate.

Family Medical Leave Act: A federal regulation that allows an employee to take time off work for a term because of a medical condition such as pregnancy and illnesses.

Food and Drug Administration (FDA): A federal agency that regulates food and drug safety for consumers. It regulates meat processing plants and other producers of foods for human consumption, and it regulates medication approval before pharmaceuticals can sold to the consumer.

Foster care homes: A prescribed physical structure that provides care and services. The number of residents served in these homes may vary from state to state but usually is considered to be a homelike setting.

Life Safety Code: Codes described by the National Fire Protection Association to provide state and local building departments guidelines for regulating building codes. These codes are usually adopted by local and state agencies, but are not mandated by the federal government.

Material Safety Data Sheets (MSDSs): Explanation of the contents of the chemical products with which an employee uses in the healthcare facility. MSDSs provide the chemical name for the product as well as the commercial name, chemical contents of the product, hazards of the product, what to do in the event of physical exposure to the product, as well as combustibility information and how to use the product safely. Can be obtained from the retailer of the product or the manufacturer.

Medical model of care: Care that focuses on the medical or disease-oriented needs of the resident and the treatment and outcome of the medical care.

National Fire Protection Association (NFPA): A national association that prescribes safety codes and definitions for state and local agencies to adopt as building regulations.

Occupational Health and Safety Administration: Federal guidelines that include safety requirements of the workplace to protect employees and reporting guidelines for illnesses, injuries, and exposure to hazardous substances that occur in the workplace.

Preventive maintenance: Proper maintenance of equipment as designated by the manufacturer to ensure the continuing functioning of equipment, safely and properly.

Residential care homes: A program approach, similar to that of an assisted living facility, that provides 24-hour housing and services. In some states, residential care and assisted living facilities are regulated by the same state rules and regulations.

Social model of care: Care that focuses on the entire person so that the resident may continue to function in a normal and accepted way.

Zoning laws: Laws established in a community that specify how buildings are to be constructed, what types of buildings may be constructed in what areas of the community, as well as established standards in building construction that ensure safety for the intended use.

REFERENCES

Allen, James. 2004 *Assisted Living Administration: The Knowledge Base.* Springer.

Buttaro, Peter. 1999 *Principles of Long Term Care.* Aspen.

Buttaro 2002 *Principles of Long Term Care— 2nd Edition.* Aspen.

Pearce, Benjamin W. 1998 *Senior Living Communities: Operations Management and Marketing for Assisted Living, Congregate, and Continuing-Care Retirement Communities.* The Johns Hopkins University Press.

Pratt, John. 2004 *Long-term Care: Managing Across the Continuum (Second Edition);* Jones and Bartlett Publishers, Inc.

Wolf, Alisa. 2002 "NFPA Standards Guide Life Safety for Many Assisted-Living Facilities." *NFPA Journal.* National Fire Protection Association.

PRACTICE QUESTIONS

1. According to OSHA, *all* employers, regardless of their size, must do which of the following?
   A. Display OSHA posters.
   B. Make reasonable accommodations.
   C. Provide employee health insurance.
   D. Establish a safety committee.

   A B C D
   ○ ○ ○ ○

2. Death by fires is mainly caused by:
   A. induced panic.
   B. faulty evacuation.
   C. severe burns.
   D. smoke inhalation.

   A B C D
   ○ ○ ○ ○

3. Which of the following would address the proper slope of an exiting wheelchair ramp?
   A. Americans with Disability Act (ADA)
   B. American Institute on Aging (AIA)
   C. National Fire Protection Agency (NFPA)
   D. Americans for Retired Citizens (ARC)

   A B C D
   ○ ○ ○ ○

4. The choice of which housekeeping services are needed is responsibility of whom?
   A. Family
   B. Resident
   C. Doctor
   D. Staff

   A B C D
   ○ ○ ○ ○

5. According to national studies, the majority of the elderly population prefer to receive care where?
   A. In the hospital
   B. In a nursing home
   C. In their own home
   D. In an assisted living center

   A B C D
   ○ ○ ○ ○

6. To ensure an RC/AL facility doesn't evolve into an institutional setting the administrator must:
   A. train new staff on the philosophy of assisted living.
   B. hire only those employees who don't come from a nursing facility.
   C. have a small number of residents.
   D. not allow nursing services.

   A B C D
   ○ ○ ○ ○

7. The best way to reduce maintenance on equipment is to:
   A. always hire outside vendors to work on equipment.
   B. have a preventive maintenance program in place.
   C. not allow staff to make any repairs.
   D. always inform the administrator of every repair.

   A B C D
   ○ ○ ○ ○

8. A facility disaster and emergency plan
   A. should be in place only when the facility is in an area where earthquakes and storms are prevalent.
   B. is for the protection of the residents and staff in case of an emergency.
   C. is provided by the local fire department.
   D. is so that residents know who will continue to care for them in a disaster.

   A B C D
   ○ ○ ○ ○

9. The social model of care focuses on which of the following factors?
   A. Personal choice and homelike environment
   B. Making sure every resident is involved in activities
   C. Residents that have special social needs
   D. In-home care services

   A B C D
   ○ ○ ○ ○

10. When a person visits an RC/AL facility, the *first impression* of a good facility and the factor that shows the person that the administrator pays attention to detail is which of the following?
    A. The upkeep of the outside grounds
    B. How happy residents are
    C. How well the meals are prepared
    D. The cleanliness of the rooms

    A B C D
    ○ ○ ○ ○

ANSWERS AND EXPLANATIONS

1. **Correct answer = A.** The other answers depend on size and type of employer or condition.
2. **Correct answer = D.** According to NFPA statistics, smoke is the greatest cause of death.
3. **Correct answer = A.** ADA deals with accessibility for persons with disabilities.
4. **Correct answer = B.** The concept of having the resident choose rather than having others make choice for the resident is important in the philosophy of assisted living.
5. **Correct answer = C.** Most individuals feel most comfortable at home and not in an institutionalized setting.
6. **Correct answer = A.** New staff need training on the philosophy of assisted living so that they do not effect an evolution of the facility into a more institutionalized setting.
7. **Correct answer = B.** Breakdown of equipment can be minimized by practicing regularly scheduled preventive maintenance.
8. **Correct answer = B.** All facilities need to develop a plan of action in case of an emergency.
9. **Correct answer = A.** The social model of care emphasizes individuality and choice in a homelike setting.
10. **Correct answer = A.** The first thing a visitor sees is the outside ground maintenance and it will create an impression as to whether the administrator pays attention to detail.

CHRISTIAN A. MASON has extensive experience in operations for assisted living communities and many other types of long term care. Prior to founding Vigilan, Chris served as chief operating officer of Sun Retirement Corporation. Chris is a founding member of the Oregon Assisted Living Facilities Association, has served on the faculty of one of the first national training programs for assisted living, has contributed to the development of the first national licensing exam, and has served as an editor of one of the first national preparatory courses for assisted living. Chris is nationally licensed and certified in assisted living and nursing home management. Chris received his MBA from Whittemore School of Business and Economics, University of New Hampshire.

CHAPTER 7

FINANCIAL MANAGEMENT

Christian A. Mason

Introduction

A residential care/assisted living (RC/AL) administrator must have broad business management knowledge to manage the complex financial nature of today's RC/AL community. Against this they must balance changing market demands and evolving service requirements.

To operate residential care/assisted living facilities successfully today, administrators need the broad general knowledge of how to manage the business financially, but must be able to delegate specific individual tasks such as keeping the books or sending out invoices. This understanding allows the administrator to keep a finger on the pulse of the community and see the big picture. It is one thing to know how to apply a **debit** or **credit**. It is a far different thing to be able to read a set of financial statements and know that there is enough cash in the bank to pay bills, meet payroll, and make money at the end of the month.

Financial management is the glue that cements together all areas of the organization and helps the administrator understand those tangible and intangible items such as census, **acuity**, turnover, regulations, personnel, cost of supplies, debt service, goodwill, and competition, all of which affect the profitability of the facility.

Overview of Domain

The National Association of Boards of Examiners of Long Term Care Administrators has established domains of practice (which determine the parameters of the NAB Residential Care/Assisted Living Examination) that highlight areas of knowledge, skill, and understanding. In the area of business/financial management are seven areas of understanding that the administrator must successfully navigate to pass this section of the licensing exam.

To *understand* the elements in this area, the administrator must be able to do the following:

1. Ensure financial management policies and practices comply with applicable federal, state, and local laws, rules, and regulations (i.e., IRS, Medicaid, Medicare, Health Insurance Portability and Accountability Act [HIPAA])
2. Ensure financial policies and procedures comply with Generally Accepted Accounting Principles (GAAP) (e.g., **accounts receivable** and payable, payroll, client/resident funds)
3. Develop, implement, and evaluate the assisted living community's **budget** (e.g., revenues, expenses, capital expenditures)
4. Develop long term projections of revenue mix and expense to ensure continued financial viability of the assisted living community
5. Monitor and comply with the assisted living community's financing obligations
6. Maintain appropriate insurance coverage to protect the assisted living community
7. Develop and implement a system to periodically monitor and adjust financial performance.

105

Map to Success

The following pages provide the candidate with a general overview of each of the areas of understanding. In those areas, the candidate will have an opportunity to review the knowledge and skill that must be gained to complete the financial/business management area of the national licensing exam successfully.

Area of Understanding I

Ensure financial management policies and practices comply with applicable federal, state, and local laws, rules, and regulations (i.e., IRS, Medicaid, Medicare, HIPAA).

Compliance with Laws, Regulations, and Rules

Administrators must comply with a large number of federal laws, regulations, and rules. Also, a number of local laws guide the management and operation of residential care and assisted living, and these laws vary by state.

Here are summaries of some of the most critical federal laws pertaining to financial management issues of residential care and assisted living.

Medicare. Medicare provides basic healthcare benefits to those over age 65, people on Social Security disability for 26 months or longer, and people with end-stage renal disease. Medicare has two parts: Part A for hospital services, and Part B that pays for home health services and hospice care for terminally ill patients. Residents in RC/AL communities who require home health or hospice services use Part B. Under Part B, services payment can be made for up to 100 home health visits provided by a home health agency for up to 12 months after the patient's discharge from a hospital or nursing home, provided certain conditions apply.

Medicare also has an anti-kickback law that penalizes anyone who knowingly and willfully solicits, receives, offers, or pays remuneration in cash or in kind to induce or in return for (1) referring an individual to a person for the furnishing or arranging for the furnishing of an item or service to be paid for by the Medicare and Medicaid program, or (2) arranging or recommending the purchase, lease, or order of goods, facility, or item to be paid for under Medicare or Medicaid.

The most significant legislative change to Medicare is the Medicare Modernization Act, or MMA, that was signed into law in December 2003. This historic legislation adds an outpatient prescription drug benefit (Part D) to Medicare; residents in RC/AL communities can use Part D coverage as well.

Medicaid. Medicaid was enacted in 1965 as an amendment to the Social Security Act of 1935 (Title XIX, 42 U.S.C.A. § 1396), entitling low-income, blind, and disabled persons to medical care. Medicaid is a vendor plan because payment is made directly to the vendor (the person or entity that provides the services) rather than to the patient. Only approved providers of medical care are entitled to receive Medicaid payments for their services. Because of skyrocketing medical expenditures, almost all states have received waivers from the federal government concerning the various elements of the Medicaid program. The federal government has also granted waivers to certain states that prefer to pay for home and community care for elderly beneficiaries who otherwise would end up in nursing homes. This type of care is less expensive than nursing home care is and allows state funds to be stretched farther. Oregon was the first state to receive a waiver to provide assisted living services in the community; there are currently 26 states that accept Medicaid waiver monies to pay for RC/AL services.

American with Disabilities Act. The Americans with Disabilities Act of 1990 prohibits discrimination based on disability. It affords similar protections against discrimination to Americans with disabilities as the Civil Rights

Act of 1964, which made discrimination based on race, religion, sex, national origin, and other characteristics illegal.

Health Insurance Portability and Accountability Act. The Health Insurance Portability and Accountability Act (HIPAA) was enacted in 1996 (45 CFR, Parts 160, 162, and 164, as amended through February 2006). According to the Centers for Medicare and Medicaid Services (CMS), Title I of HIPAA protects health insurance coverage for workers and their families when they change or lose their jobs. Title II of HIPAA, the Administrative Simplification provisions, requires the establishment of national standards for electronic healthcare transactions and national identifiers for providers, health insurance plans, and employers.

Privacy provision. The HIPAA privacy provision took effect on April 14, 2003, with a one-year extension for certain "small plans."

Key privacy provisions include the following:

- Individuals must be able to access their record and request correction of errors.
- Individuals must be informed of how their personal information will be used.
- Individuals' protected health information cannot be used for marketing purposes without the explicit consent of the involved individuals.
- Individuals can ask covered entities that maintain protected health information about them to take reasonable steps to ensure that their communications with the individual are confidential.
- Individuals can file formal privacy-related complaints to the Department of Health and Human Services (HHS) Office for Civil Rights.
- Covered entities must document their privacy procedures.
- Covered entities must designate a privacy officer and train their employees.
- Covered entities may use an individual's information without the individual's consent for the purposes of providing treatment, obtaining payment for services, and performing the nontreatment operational tasks of the provider's business.

HIPAA Electronic Data Interchange (HIPAA/EDI). The HIPAA/EDI provision was scheduled to take effect October 16, 2003, with a one-year extension for certain "small plans"; however, because of widespread confusion and difficulty in implementing the rule, CMS granted a one-year extension to all parties. As of October 16, 2004, full implementation was not achieved and CMS began an open-ended "contingency period." Penalties for noncompliance were not levied; however, all parties are expected to make a "good-faith effort" to come into compliance. CMS ended the Medicare contingency period July 1, 2005. Today, to be paid most medical providers must file their electronic claims using the HIPAA standards. There are exceptions for doctors that meet certain criteria.

Sarbanes-Oxley. The Sarbanes-Oxley Act of 2002 deals with truth in financial reporting. This law established a Public Company Accounting Oversight Board (PCAOB), which operates under the Securities and Exchange Commission (SEC). Sarbanes-Oxley requires companies to report on their finances and be checked by independent auditors. A key element of Sarbanes-Oxley is that companies must monitor and report on their company's internal controls. Internal controls are actions and policies that a company uses to achieve goals, especially in the financial realm. Sarbanes-Oxley makes it necessary for them to watch and document both the methods used and the results produced. Additionally, Sarbanes-Oxley requires companies to submit an annual assessment of their effectiveness of internal **auditing** to the SEC.

Most important, Sarbanes-Oxley places responsibility on the shoulders of executives. Corporate CEOs and CFOs must review and sign off on financial audits. Sarbanes-Oxley holds executives responsible with both civil and criminal penalties.

Area of Understanding II

Ensure financial policies and procedures comply with Generally Accepted Accounting Principles (GAAP) (e.g., accounts receivable and payable, payroll, client/resident funds).

Generally Accepted Accounting Principles

The Generally Accepted Accounting Principles (GAAP) are a widely accepted set of rules, conventions, standards, and procedures for reporting financial information, as established by the Financial Accounting Standards Board (FASB; Statement of Auditing Standards [SAS] No. 91).

GAAP standards are imposed on organizations so that investors have a minimum level of consistency in the financial statements they use when analyzing companies for investment purposes. GAAP covers such things as revenue recognition, balance sheet item classification, and outstanding share measurements.

Companies are expected to follow GAAP rules when reporting their financial data via financial statements. These financial statements represent a company's annual statement of financial operations. Annual reports include a balance sheet, income statement, statement of change in financial position, auditor's report, and a description of the company's operations.

The accrual accounting method measures the performance and position of a company by recognizing economic events regardless of when cash transactions occur. This method allows the current cash inflows/outflows to be combined with future expected cash inflows/outflows to give a more accurate picture of a company's current financial condition (Allen 2005).

Accrual accounting is considered to be the standard accounting practice for most residential care and assisted living companies. This method provides a more accurate picture of the company's current condition, but its relative complexity makes it more expensive to implement. This is the opposite of cash accounting, which recognizes transactions only when there is an exchange of cash.

When we examine the accounting practices of residential care/assisted living communities, we must also examine the differences between for-profit organizations and not-for-profit organizations to understand how information is tracked and recorded.

Differences Between Not-for-Profit and For-Profit Accounting

The two primary differences between for-profit organizations and not-for-profit organizations are (1) not-for-profit organizations are mission-based rather than existing for the financial benefit of owners or shareholders, and (2) most not-for-profits receive a portion of their income from contributions.

Not-for-profit organizations break down expenses on both a line item basis (such as salaries or food) as well as by functional categories (such as programs and fund-raising) (Hawkins 2004).

Gifts, donations, endowments, and other forms of contributed income also differentiate not-for-profits from for-profits. The general rules for accounting for contributions in not-for-profits are to ensure that donations will be used as the donor intended. To do this, not-for-profits must record contributions in one of the following categories: unrestricted, temporarily restricted, or permanently restricted.

Unrestricted gifts and donations may be included in general income and used for the general benefit of the organization. The donor has made the contribution without specifying a purpose or time period within which the funds must be used.

Temporarily restricted funds are those that are donated for a specific purpose or for use during a specific period of time. Not-for-profits are required to track the balances of these gifts separately from unrestricted ones.

Permanently restricted contributions most often take the form of endowments. Typically, this means that organizations can invest the funds to generate income, but they are not allowed to spend the original contributions.

These two differences between not-for-profits and for-profits (tracking expenses by function and tracking contributions by level of restriction) result in not-for-profit organizations having financial statements that are somewhat different from for-profit enterprises (Moore 2003).

Financial Statement Analysis

Readers of financial statements can learn a great deal about the health of an organization by examining the numerical information presented. Key financial statements include the following:

- Balance sheet—a financial snapshot of an organization at one point in time
- Income statement or statement of operations—a measure of financial flows over time
- Cash flow statement—aggregate data regarding all cash inflows and cash outflows (cash flow statements are covered in more detail later in this chapter)

In many cases, ratio analysis is used to evaluate an organization's financial health. The ratios used to evaluate for-profit organizations versus not-for-profit organizations differ in some cases. Ratios are a tool for comparing numbers representing different aspects of an organization's financial health.

Income Statement or Statement of Operations

In for-profit organizations, the **income statement** is a financial report that summarizes revenues and expenses and shows the net profit or loss for a specified **accounting period**. This financial report is also known as the *profit and loss statement* or *statement of revenue and expense*. The income statement is the most analyzed portion of the financial statements. It displays how well the company can ensure success for both itself

and its shareholders through the earnings from operations.

In not-for-profit organizations, the financial report that summarizes this information is referred to as the statement of operations. Financial indicators from this statement include the following:

- *Surplus or deficit.* If income is greater than expenses in a given period, say a year, the organization has generated a surplus. If expenses are greater than revenue, the organization experiences a deficit for the period. In a for-profit organization, a deficit indicates a loss and is viewed as a negative financial indicator. In not-for-profit organizations, there is no rule indicating an organization should have surpluses, deficits, or break even. Typically, not-for-profits budget to break even. However, organization may deliberately decide to spend down their cash reserves (expandable net **assets**) for a specific purpose such as funding a new program. Doing so may result in a planned operating deficit. Similarly, if a not-for-profit has determined that it needs to build cash reserves for future mission-driven purposes, it may reflect a surplus.
- *Budget to actual for revenue and expense.* Perhaps the most commonly used financial indicator is a comparison of budgeted revenue to actual revenue, and budgeted expense to actual expense. These comparisons are made on both a monthly and a year-to-date basis. Variations from budget are analyzed and described as variances. This type of analysis is common to both for-profit and not-for-profit organizations.
- *Net operating income margin.* This is defined as:

$$\frac{\textbf{Operating Expenses}}{\textbf{Total Revenue}}$$

109

This ratio indicates what the company's pricing policy is and what its true operating margins are. This is very useful when comparing against the margins of previous years. This is used to calculate operating margins for the total community.

- *Functional expense ratios (nonprofit).* When completing Federal Form 900, not-for-profits must report expenses functionally, broken down into the categories of Program, Management and General Activities, and Fund-raising.
- *Program expense divided by total expense.* If high, most of the expenses are related to program. This may mean that little is spent on management or on fund-raising.
- *Fund-raising expense divided by total expense.* If high, a large percentage of expenses are spent on fund-raising efforts. Prospective donors may draw the conclusion that too much is being spent on fund-raising and not enough on program services.
- *Interest coverage.* This is defined as:

$$\frac{\text{EBITDA}}{\text{Interest Expense}}$$

This ratio indicates what portion of debt interest is covered by a company's cash flow situation. An interest coverage ratio under 1 means a community is having problems generating enough cash flow to pay interest expense. Ideally, you want the ratio to be over 1.5. EBITDA stands for *earnings before interest taxes depreciation and amortization.* A related acronym, EBITDAR, means the same thing, but the *R* includes deferred taxes.

Balance Sheet or Statement of Position

In the for-profit arena, the **balance sheet** is the financial statement that summarizes a company's assets, **liabilities**, and shareholders' **equity** at a specific point in time. The three balance sheet segments give owners, investors, and other stakeholders a summary of what the company owns and owes, as well as the amount invested by the shareholders (Allen 2005).

The balance sheet must follow the following formula:

$$\textbf{Assets} = \textbf{Liabilities} + \textbf{Shareholders' Equity}$$

The three segments of the balance sheet contain many numbered **accounts** that document current values. Accounts such as cash, accounts receivable, and prepaid items are on the asset side of the balance sheet, while on the liability side there are accounts such as **accounts payable**, short-term debt, and long-term debt. The exact accounts on a balance sheet differ by company and by industry.

It is called a balance sheet because the two sides balance out. This makes sense: a company has to pay for all the things it has (assets) by either borrowing money (liabilities) or getting it from shareholders (shareholders' equity).

The **balance sheet** is one of the most important pieces of financial information issued by a company. It is a snapshot of what a company owns and owes at that point in time. The income statement, on the other hand, shows how much revenue and profit a company has generated over a certain period. Neither statement is better than the other—rather, the financial statements are built to be used together to present a complete picture of a company's finances.

In the not-for-profit arena, this financial statement is known as the **statement of financial position**. Whereas the statement of activities depicts the overall status of your profits (or deficits) by looking at income and expenses over a period of time, the balance sheet depicts the overall status of your finances at a fixed point in time. It totals all your assets and subtracts all your liabilities to compute your overall **net worth** (or net loss). This statement is referenced particularly when applying for funding.

Financial indicators from the balance sheet or statement of financial position include the following:

- *Short-term liabilities coverage ratio or Acid Test (quick ratio).* Will there be enough cash to pay bills in the near future? Add all assets that can be used to pay bills over a specific period of time and compare this with the bills that must be paid in that same period of time (Allen 2005).

  For a not-for-profit: This is generally calculated by Cash + Unrestricted Investment + Accounts Receivable divided by Current Accounts Payable + Current Accruals.

  For a for-profit: This is generally calculated by Cash + Accounts Receivable + Short-term Investments divided by Current Liabilities.

  This ratio provides a stringent test that indicates if a firm has enough short-term assets to cover its immediate liabilities. It is similar but a more strenuous version of the working capital ratio, indicating whether liabilities could be paid without selling other assets.

- *Working capital or current ratio.* Will cash flow be adequate to pay bills over the next year? Look at:

$$\frac{\textbf{Current Assets}}{\textbf{Current Liabilities}}$$

  This ratio indicates if a firm has enough short-term assets to cover its immediate liabilities. If the ratio is less than 1, the firm has negative **working capital**. Caution: Even if **current ratio** is adequately calculated for the year, there may be periods in the year when there is an inadequate cash flow to pay bills (Allen 2005).

- *Solvency ratio.* This is one of many ratios used to gauge a company's ability to meet long term obligations. Taking a company's net worth and dividing by total assets derives this ratio.

- *Deferred revenue or net temporarily restricted assets (nonprofit).* Deferred revenue traditionally refers to cash that has been received for some restricted condition that has not yet been met. Under the new Statement of Financial Accounting Standards No.116 issued by the Financial Accounting Standards Board (FASB), most of these funds will be held not as deferred revenue, but as an addition to temporarily restricted net assets.

  To determine the ratio, take the Deferred Revenue (temporarily restricted net assets) and divide by the Cash + Savings. If deferred revenue or temporarily restricted net assets exceeds cash and savings, you may be spending restricted cash for purposes other than those that the funds were intended.

- *Average interest rate.* This is:

$$\frac{\textbf{Accounts Payable}}{\textbf{Liabilities}}$$

  This ratio indicates the average interest rate that a community must pay to service its debt.

- *Return on equity—ROE (for profit).* This is:

$$\frac{\textbf{Net Income}}{\textbf{Owners' Equity}}$$

  This ratio indicates what return a community is generating on the owners' investment. Averaging ROE over the past 5 to 10 years can give you a better idea of historical growth.

- *Asset turnover.* This is:

$$\frac{\textbf{Revenue}}{\textbf{Total Assets}}$$

  This ratio indicates the relationship between assets and revenue.

- *Collection ratio.* This is:

$$\frac{\textbf{Accounts Receivable}}{\textbf{(Revenue / 365)}}$$

This ratio indicates the average number of days it takes a company to collect unpaid invoices. A high ratio indicates that the company is having problems getting paid for services or products.

- *Debt–asset ratio.* This is:

Total Liabilities
Total Assets

This ratio indicates what proportions of the company's assets are being financed through debt. This ratio is very similar to the debt–equity ratio. A ratio under 1 means a majority of assets is financed through equity.

Cash Flow or Statement of Change in Financial Position

The cash flow statement or statement of change in financial position is a document providing aggregate data regarding all cash inflows a company receives from both its ongoing operations and external investment sources, as well as all cash outflows that pay for business activities and investments during a given period of time.

To have a positive cash flow, the company's long term cash inflows need to exceed its long term cash outflows. An outflow of cash occurs when a company transfers funds to another party. Such a transfer could be made to pay for employees, suppliers, and creditors or to purchase long term assets and investments.

A cash inflow is of course the exact opposite; it is any transfer of money that comes into the company's possession. Typically, the majority of a company's cash inflows are from customers, lenders, and investors. Occasionally, cash flows come from sources such as legal settlements or the sale of company real estate or equipment.

It is important to note the distinction between being profitable and having positive cash flow transactions: just because an assisted living community is bringing in cash does not mean it is making a profit.

For example, say an assisted living community is experiencing low census and therefore decides to sell off the community vehicle. It will receive cash from the buyer for the used vehicle. In the month that it sold the vehicle, the community would end up with a strong positive cash flow, but its current and future earnings potential would still be fairly bleak. Because cash flow can be positive while profitability is negative, administrators should analyze income statements as well as cash flow statements, not just one or the other.

Because companies tend to use accrual accounting, the income statements may not necessarily reflect changes in their cash positions. For example, an assisted living facility needs to put on a new roof. The cost of the roof would be capitalized and only a small portion of the cost would be shown on the income statement as **depreciation**, but the company must pay the full price of the roof at the time the job is completed. While the facility may be earning a profit (and paying income taxes on it), the facility may, during the quarter, actually end up with less cash than when it started the quarter. Even profitable facilities can fail to adequately manage their cash flow, which is why the cash flow statement is important: it helps stakeholders see if a facility is having trouble with cash.

The balance sheet gives a one-time snapshot of a company's assets and liabilities, and the income statement indicates the business's profitability during a certain period. The cash flow statement acts as a kind of corporate checkbook that reconciles the other two statements. The cash flow statement generally shows cash flows in and out of the organization in three areas. These include cash flow from operating activities, cash flows from investing activities, and cash flows from financing activities.

Cash flows from operating activities include the revenues and expenses of the day-to-day operations of the organization. Cash flows from investing would include dollars earned or spent in investment activities such as money earned on money market funds from surplus revenues deposited. Cash flow from financing would include items such as the cost of capital to refinance a loan or piece of capital equipment.

Financial Indicators Using Information from Multiple Financial Statements

Fund balance ratio or unrestricted net assets ratio (nonprofit). The fund balance ratio, now called the unrestricted net assets ratio, measures the amount of unrestricted, expendable equity to the organization's annual operating expense. To determine the ratio, use this equation:

$$\frac{\textbf{Expendable Unrestricted Net Assets}}{\textbf{Annual Expenses}}$$

A low number indicates an organization has little unrestricted, expendable equity available to meet temporary cash shortages or deficit situations in the future.

Service quotient. This is:

$$\frac{\textbf{Service Revenue}}{\textbf{Service Cost}}$$

This ratio determines whether care services provided by the assisted living community are profitable or whether they are being subsidized by other charges. Service revenues are dollars received by the assisted living community for care delivered by nursing staff. Service costs are the total labor costs for direct care staff and nursing. This number should include the fully loaded cost of care (i.e., cost of benefits). If the service quotient is less than 1, services are being delivered at a loss.

Valuation

According to the Appraisal Institute, valuation is a method used to convert a single year's income expectancy into an indication of value in one direct step, by dividing the income estimate by an appropriate rate.

This rate is known as the cap rate. The relationship between cap rate (R), income (I), and estimated value (V) is:

$$\textbf{Value} = \frac{\textbf{Income}}{\textbf{Rate}}$$

Internal Control

Internal accounting control is a series of procedures designed to provide sound management and financial practices. Following internal accounting control procedures will significantly increase the likelihood of the following:

- Financial information is reliable.
- Assets and records of the organization are properly managed and maintained.
- The organization's policies are followed.
- Proper accounting rules are followed.

Developing an Internal Accounting Control System

The first step in developing an effective internal accounting control system is to identify those areas where problems or errors may occur. Elements of an effective internal accounting control system include well-defined policy and procedures for managing the following accounting systems:

- *Cash receipts.* Ensure that all cash intended for the organization is received, promptly deposited, properly recorded, reconciled, and kept under adequate security.
- *Cash disbursements.* Ensure that cash is disbursed only upon proper authorization of management, for valid business purposes, and that all disbursements are properly recorded.
- *Petty cash.* Ensure that petty cash and other working funds are disbursed only for proper purposes, are adequately safeguarded, and are properly recorded.
- *Payroll.* Ensure that payroll disbursements are made only upon proper authorization to bona fide employees, that payroll disbursements are properly

113

recorded, and that related legal requirements (such as payroll tax deposits) are complied with.

- *Grants, gifts, and bequests.* Ensure that all grants, gifts, and bequests are received and properly recorded and that compliance with the terms of any related restrictions is adequately monitored.
- *Fixed assets.* Ensure that **fixed assets** are acquired and disposed of only upon proper authorization, are adequately safeguarded, and are properly recorded.

The most important concept in developing good internal control procedures is segregation of duties. It is important to distribute duties and tasks so as to not leave control for the management of resources in the hands of a single individual. An example of where segregation of duties is critical is in the issuance of checks. The person signing the check should not be the same person authorizing payment.

The policies and procedures for handling financial transactions are best recorded in an Accounting Policies and Procedures Manual. This manual can be used to describe the administrative tasks and who is responsible for each. The executive director or administrator is commonly responsible for overseeing the day-to-day implementation of these policies and procedures.

The auditor's management letter is an important indicator of the adequacy of your internal accounting control structure, and the degree to which it is maintained. The management letter, which accompanies the audit and is typically addressed to the board as trustees or the ownership of the organization, cites significant weaknesses in the system or its execution. By reviewing the management letter with the executive director, asking for responses to each internal control lapse or recommendation, and comparing management letters from year to year, the board has a useful mechanism for monitoring its financial safeguards and adherence to financial policies (Hawkins 2004).

Area of Understanding III

Develop, implement, and evaluate the assisted living community's budget (e.g., revenues, expenses, capital expenditures).

Budgeting

Financial management is the integration and reporting of financial information that results from the operation of interlocking **control systems** designed to manage and measure an organization's success.

Financial management encompasses planning, directing, evaluating, and monitoring all the facility's management systems that affect revenues and expenses. The administrator's role is to balance the many aspects of financial management by providing clear oversight for the many interlocking systems and controls that involve the various internal and external components. Financial management is an administrative function, which differentiates it from the role of a financial officer. When an administrator begins to examine the process of budgeting, he or she must first be aware of the different types of budgets used by the facility and how each are interrelated. In today's residential care/assisted living facility, an administrator is charged with the oversight of all budgeting activities related to the community.

Common terms administrators will encounter in building budgets include the following:

- *Operating budget.* An itemized forecast of a company's income and expenses expected for some period in the future.
- *Capital budget.* Plan to finance long term outlays, such as for fixed assets like facilities and equipment. *Capital* is money invested in the facility. In general terms, capital budgets are typically used for items that cost in excess of $500 and have a minimum useful life of longer than one year. (Items with a useful life of less than one year would usually be expensed.) In practice, however, different companies

have different thresholds that could be lower or higher than $500.

- *Development budget.* A plan to determine the resources, timeline, and budget to complete a project.
- *Construction budget.* Budgets used to determine the hard and soft costs related to the construction of new communities. Hard costs include land and construction costs. Soft costs include items such as insurance, engineering, and architectural, development costs.
- *Acquisition budgets.* An accounting method used in mergers and acquisitions with which the purchasing company treats the target firm as an investment, adding the target's assets to its own fair market value. If the amount paid for a company is greater than fair market value, the difference is reflected as goodwill. Because goodwill must be written off against future earnings, this makes the pooling-of-interests method preferable.
- *Fixed budget.* A fixed budget is one that is made without regard to potential variations in business activity. This type of budgeting is effective for companies with low variable costs.
- *Activity-based budgeting:* A method of budgeting in which activities that incur costs in each function of an organization are established and relationships are defined between activities. This information is then used to decide how much resource should be allocated to each activity.

A method of budgeting in which all expenditures must be justified each new period, as opposed to only explaining the amounts requested in excess of the previous period's funding.

- *Zero-based budgeting.* If an organization uses zero-based budgets, each department must justify its funding every year. That is, funding has a base at zero. A department must show why its funding

efficiently helps the organization toward its goals.

Zero-based budgeting is especially encouraged for government budgets because expenditures can easily run out of control if it is automatically assumed what was spent last year must be spent this year. (Allen 2005)

To many, a budget is simply an estimation of the revenue and expenses over a specified future period of time for an organization or business entity. Budgets show the financial trade-off made when one good is exchanged for another (Allen 2005).

A budget surplus means profits are anticipated; a balanced budget means revenues are expected to equal expenses; and a deficit budget means expenses will exceed revenue. Budgets are usually compiled and reevaluated on a periodic basis. Adjustments are made to budgets based on the goals of the budgeting organization.

Most operating budgets are built from the top down. They begin with an analysis of revenues, and then match expenses to available resources. The administrator is responsible for developing a facility's revenue projection based upon available revenue sources. The administrator must analyze historic performance and project future opportunity.

In developing an operating budget for a community, an administrator should keep in mind the following ideas regarding the creation of a budget.

1. Provide a means by which resources are allocated.
2. Provide a road map for the organization to navigate into the future.
3. Tell the story of the organization: where have we come from and where are we going?
4. Provide a framework for benchmarking decisions.
5. Help measure success.

Key elements of most operating budgets include a set of assumptions regarding the current and expected future state of the business. These are usually the key variables that you will build your financial model on. These include the following:

- An analysis of current room rates, market rates, and vacancy rates by unit.
- An analysis of expected revenue to be produced by the community. This includes rents, ancillary revenue, as well as service revenues
- Investment summary (a summary of the overall return to investors based on the performance of the community)
- Budget summary (a summary of key consolidated revenues and expenses by area. Revenues are generally by type and expenses are generally summarized by area of operation).
- Staff hours summary (a summary of staffing hours by area of operation).
- Staff dollars summary (a summary of **salary** and **wages** by area with annual increases and benefits factored in).
- Census analysis (an analysis of census and occupancy by unit type and actual unit).
- Marketing data analysis (an analysis of inquiries, tours, deposits, move ins and move outs for the community).
- Staff turnover analysis (an analysis of staff change by position throughout the previous year. This includes terminations, discharges, and resignations).
- Capital needs analysis (an analysis of the capital replacement requirements for the community. Capital budgets are used to maintain, replace, or upgrade the assets of the business).

Some of the common terms used in budgeting include **chart of accounts**; profit margin; cash flow; earnings before interest taxes, depreciation, and **amortization** (EBITDAR); acuity; variable and fixed costs; direct and indirect costs; revenue mix; turnover; wage rates; and payment mix. These terms are explained in the following list.

- *Chart of accounts.* The chart of accounts is a list of every account in the facility. The accounts are organized into five groups:
  - Assets—things owned by the facility
  - Liabilities—obligations of the facility
  - Capital—money invested in the facility
  - Revenues—earnings from operations and investments
  - Expenses—cost of salaries, supplies, and so forth that have been used up through the provision of service

  There is also a sixth group for nonprofit organizations: fund accounts. Fund accounts include all funds established for restricted or unrestricted use (Allen 2005).
- *Profit margin.* Profit margin is defined as the ratio of income to sales. There are two types of profit margin: gross profit margin and net profit margin. Gross profit margin shows the percentage return that the facility is earning over the cost of providing services. It is defined as gross profit divided by sales. Net profit shows the percentage of net income generated by each service in for-profit facilities. It is defined as net income divided by sales (Allen 2005). This ratio indicates what portions of revenues contribute to the income of a community. A low profit margin can indicate pricing strategy and/or the impact competition has on margins.
- *Cash flow.* Cash flow is the cash receipts less the cash disbursements from a given operation or set of operations for a specific period of time (Allen 2005).
- *Depreciation.* Depreciable assets are those used to provide services during more than one time period; in the course of operations, they use value as a result of use, wear and tear, or obsolescence (Allen 2005). It is important to remember that depreciable assets are used in the facility operations. Depreciation is also a process by which the cost of an

asset is spread over its useful life. In most organizations, a minimum dollar amount such as $200 is used to set the floor for depreciating the asset.

- *EBITDAR.* This term is used to define net income plus depreciation and amortization plus deferred taxes.
- *Acuity.* A measure of resident need or want using numerical or time-based scoring to measure the level of care required in the activities of daily living (ADL) and instrumental activities of daily living (IADL) assistance categories.
- *Variable cost.* Variable costs are those that fluctuate directly and proportionately with changes in volume.
- *Fixed cost.* These are costs that do not relate to changes in volume. The cost of the administrator's salary will not change based on the number of residents in the community.
- *Direct cost.* Direct costs are costs directly attributable to a revenue center or providing resident care. This usually includes all healthcare salaries, payroll, taxes, benefits, supplies, and expenses associated with capital equipment used within a department.
- *Indirect cost.* Indirect costs are costs that cannot be directly associated with a revenue-producing center, yet support the functions of the community. These include administrative salaries, depreciation, taxes, and so forth.
- *Revenue mix.* The revenue mix is the composition of revenues from the various payment sources for the community.
- *Turnover.* Turnover is a measure that indicates what percentage of a population is new during a specific timeframe, and applies both to residents and employees. (In other words, a particular facility might have had a resident turnover rate of 10 percent for the month of July—meaning that 10 percent of its residents were new that month.)

- *Wage rates.* Wage rates refer to the prevailing hourly wage for specific jobs in a geographic area.
- *Payment mix.* The payment mix is the composition of payments from various sources, with each source usually shown as a percentage of total payments.

Allen (2005) outlines five steps to the budgeting process:

1. Assessing the environment
2. Programming
3. Developing the operating budget
4. Building the cash budget
5. Determining the capital budget

The initial step in the budgeting process is to assess the external and internal environments. This includes evaluations of competition, reimbursement, regulations, economic swings, inflation, wage rates, availability of personnel, and needs of the resident population.

In the programming step, the administrator uses the information gathered to build a set of assumptions around which the budgeting process will flow. The completed budgeting process results in four types of budgets being developed, including the operating budget, the cash budget, the capital budget, and the pro forma financial statements.

During the development of the operating budget, ongoing and one-time expenses are evaluated and captured and measured against operating and nonoperating revenues.

Following the creation of an operating budget, the administrator needs to prepare a cash budget. As its name indicates, the cash budget is based on the revenues and expenses from the operating budget. The cash budget is an estimate of the cash inflows and outflows for the next 12 months, enabling the administrator to identify months with possible cash shortages and overages.

117

The final budget to be created is the capital budget. This budget reflects all anticipated capital needs (items with a life of more than 12 months) in a budget year.

In capital budgeting, a number of different approaches can be used to evaluate any given project, and each approach has its own distinct advantages and disadvantages. Furthermore, every project is unique. The particular risk and reward characteristics of a given project usually lead to one method being selected over another.

See Appendix 7.A for additional information on net present value, internal rate of return and discounted cash flow.

Area of Understanding IV

Develop long term projections of revenue mix and expense to ensure continued financial viability of the assisted living community.

Revenue

Revenue is defined as dollars earned from fees collected, products and/or services sold, and income earned from investments. Most revenue in assisted living facilities comes from rent and services provided.

Rent revenue represents fees charged for general lodging, utilities, and basic hospitality services such as meals and housekeeping.

Service revenue represents fees charged from delivery of additional care or support above a stated base rate. Service revenue sources include items such as guest meals, transportation, beauty salons, cable television, and phone services.

Payment sources include private pay, Medicaid, health maintenance organizations, and private insurance. The majority of all payments for residential care/assisted living in the United States come from private-pay sources.

To accurately forecast revenues an administrator must understand current market conditions, census patterns and trends, resident acuity (care needs), turnover, regulatory restrictions, and competition. Resident acuity often drives resident turnover and census trends. A facility with high resident acuity will likely have higher turnover than one with low acuity has. New competition in the marketplace from other assisted living communities and new emerging alternatives also play a role in forecasting revenues. The expression that revenue drives operations helps you understand the importance a facility's occupancy has on its success. Nearly as important is the manner in which a facility manages its service revenue.

Today, there are three prevailing methods for managing service revenue. The first is to combine service revenues with rental revenue for single fixed price. A second method is to charge for care based on a number of levels of care. Under this approach, residents pay an additional fee based on services needed. Services are grouped together and priced as levels. The higher the level, the more services needed and the higher the service charge. The third method is to charge on an à la carte or fee-for-service basis. This approach charges for services based on individual needs and is most often based on time. Residents choose services needed or wanted and are then charged based on the consumption of services (Moore 2004).

Example 1. In this first example, residents are charged a flat rate for rent and services delivered. This model charges all residents the same amount no matter how their individual care needs may be different.

Number of Residents	Rental Price	Total Charge
50	$2,500	$125,000

Example 2: Levels of care. Happy Assisted Living has developed a revenue model that charges for care services based on three levels of care.

Levels of Care	Care Included	Price Charged	Number of Residents	Service Revenue	Rent	Total Charge
Level 1	Dressing, ambulation, bathing	$250	10	$2,500	$20,000	$22,500
Level 2	Meds management, toileting, bowel and bladder care	$500	15	$7,500	$30,000	$37,500
Level 3	Feeding, nursing services, and nighttime checks	$750	20	$15,000	$40,000	$55,000
No Care Needs		$0	5		$10,000	$10,000
Total			50	$25,000	$100,000	$125,000
Rent	50 at $2,000 ea.					

In this example, you can see that residents are charged for care under three levels. There are a total of 45 residents receiving care services and the community is collecting a total of $25,000 in monthly service revenues. This method of charging for service does not link to staffing, care needs are not mutually exclusive, and residents often wind up receiving services from multiple levels.

Example 3: Points or units of time. In this example, residents are charged for care based on the amount of time needed on an individual basis. Residents are only charged for services needed. Facility staffing is based on the total amount of time required as calculated by adding up all of the care time identified.

Unit of Measure for Care Services	Care Included	Price Charged per Point	Number of Residents	Total Number of Points (All Residents)	Total Charge
Services 1 point = 5 minutes of care	All services have been defined in units of time equaling a set number of points	$50	50	1000	$50,000
Base Rent	$2,000 per month		50		$100,000
Total Revenues					$150,000

Revenue projections are based on average census. For example: A 50-unit assisted living facility running at 90 percent occupancy would likely have 45 units occupied at any point in time. If the average rent per unit is $2,000 and the typical service revenue is $200 per resident, the community would generate the following revenues:

Revenue	Units	Occupied	Units	Average $	Monthly
Rent	50	45	$2,000	$90,000	Rental Revenue
Services		45	$200	$9,000	Service Revenue
Total				$99,000	Total Revenue

Revenues collected in not-for-profit organizations are viewed and handled slightly differently. In addition to the sources of revenue mentioned earlier, not-for-profit organizations also receive revenues in the form of pledges, gifts, donated materials and service, and from memberships or buy-in fees.

Most revenues received by not-for-profit organizations are handled in the same manner as for-profit organizations with a few exceptions. Not-for-profits that qualify for tax-exempt status under section 501(c) (3) of the Internal Revenue Code are entitled to receive contributions that are tax deductible to the donor. Different procedures have been established for handling the following types of contributions: pledges, donated materials or services, and special events and membership dues.

In addition, the accounting profession has established guidelines for responsibly tracking monies that have been restricted by the donor for a specific use (e.g., buying a new building, starting a new program, adding to the endowment). How these monies are tracked and reported depends on the nature of the donor's restriction.

Expenses

Effectively managing costs over time requires that the administrator understands the relationship between revenues and expenses. If a facility's expenses exceed its revenues over an extended period of time, without the infusion of new capital the community will cease to be a viable economic entity.

Breakeven analysis is a method of comparing revenues and expense that helps the administrator understand the point at which available cash from operations is equal to zero. To understand this approach, two terms discussed earlier must be used, including (1) variable cost, (2) fixed cost, and a new term (3) semivariable cost.

Semivariable costs do not fit neatly into either the fixed or variable categories because they vary disproportionately with volume. Examples of semivariable costs might be total healthcare aide salaries, which depend more on resident volume and resident level of care needs than does the resident care coordinator's salary, which does not fluctuate directly with these variables (Allen 2005, 252).

While total variable costs (TVC) change with volume, the variable cost per unit does not change. Inversely, total fixed cost (TFC) does vary per unit with the change in volume. To understand these concepts, look at meal costs and administrators' salaries.

Let's first look at total variable cost (TVC). The total dollars spent on preparing a meal for the community for will depend on the number of residents eating. If the cost to prepare each meal is $3.00 and the facility prepares 100 meals, the total food cost is $300. The cost to prepare each individual meal is $3.00. The total food cost, however, changes based on the volume (number) of meals prepared.

Now let's look at total fixed cost (TFC). An administrator is paid an annual salary of $50,000 and is responsible for overseeing a 100-unit assisted living community. Based on this information, we could say the administrator's cost per resident is $500. If the number of residents increased from 100 to 200, the administrator's cost per resident would drop to $250. In this case, the cost per unit will vary with volume.

For our discussion, we can use the following equation to determine the volume of service units required to break even:

Total Fixed Cost + Total Variable Cost = Total Cost

To break even, total cost (TC) must be equal to total revenue (TR). We can substitute this information into the preceding example with the following:

**Breakeven Point means:
Total Cost = Total Revenue**

If a facility spends $10,000 a month providing care services for the nursing department, and the total fixed costs are $5,000 and the variable cost per hour of care delivered is $18.00, we can use the following approach to determine the **breakeven point** for the nursing department as follows:

$$\$10,000 = \$5,000 + (\$18 \times \text{number of care hours delivered})$$
$$\text{Number of care hours delivered} = (\$10,000 - \$5,000) / \$18$$

Nursing department breakeven (number of billable hours) point $= (\$5,000/\$18)$
Number of care hours billed
$=$ approximately 277.75

This example assumes that the RN's (director of care) salary is a fixed portion of the department's cost. In the marketplace today, many facilities are treating all nursing costs as variable and seeking to recover these costs.

One of the most important reasons for gathering this cost information is to help the administrator in setting rates for services. After the fixed and variable costs of each area of the operation are determined, the average cost per unit of service for each of those areas can be determined. We often refer to these costs as average cost per resident day (PRD) cost. You will generally see this information calculated for each department in the facility. Summarizing these costs allows the administrator to understand what service volumes and fees for service need to be charged to operate above a breakeven level.

Not-for-profits report their expenses by functional expense classification. The two primary functional expense classifications are program services and supporting activities. Supporting activities typically include management and general activities, fund-raising, and membership development. Practices vary widely from organization to organization in the nonprofit sector as to how expenses are categorized by functional areas. These costs can also be broken down into fixed and variable amounts. The process of rate setting in a not-for-profit generally includes the impact fund-raising, gifts, and endowments have in reducing average costs.

Area of Understanding V

Monitor and comply with the assisted living community's financing obligations.

The financial obligations of an assisted living community include all needs for cash. These obligations are both short and long term in nature. They arise whenever cash is needed and not available from operations or reserves.

Typically, when a community is purchased or built, a mortgage is taken out to cover the cost of building and equipment. This cost is then amortized over the expected life of the asset and paid out of operations on a monthly basis. Debt service is based on the amount financed. This may range from 70 percent to as much as 95 percent of the value of the asset.

Example: A new assisted living community is built in Salem, Oregon. The 50-unit project's total cost of construction, including all soft costs and furniture, fixtures, and equipment, is $5,000,000. The owners have received a loan for a mortgage from First Community Bank for 80 percent of the finished appraised value of the community or $4,000,000. This works out to a loan of $80,000 per unit. The loan is repayable over 30 years and contains an interest rate of 7 percent. Payments on the loan are generated from surplus cash from operating the community. The community has an obligation to make monthly payments of approximately $26,457. These payments include the repayment of both principal and interest. Most lenders require a minimum debt coverage ratio of 1.1 on a project to make the loan. In this case, the community would need to have surplus cash from operations of $26,457 × 1.1 or $29,103 to qualify for this loan.

Mortgages are typically amortized over the life of the loan. This means that the monthly cost is usually the same each month. Depreciation and amortization schedules are

New Assisted Living—Salem, Oregon		Number of Units = 50	
Construction Cost	$5,000,000	Loan from First Community Bank	$4,000,000
Cost per Unit	$100,000	Loan per Unit	$80,000
Value at Completion	$5,000,000	Loan Term	30 Years
Debt Coverage Req.	1.1	Loan Interest Rate	7%
Minimum Available Cash Requirement	$29,103	Monthly Interest and Principal Payment	$26,457

designed so that the borrower repays a level amount on a month-to-month basis rather that having to pay a fixed amount of principal, plus interest, each month. The amortization payment allows for budgeting and easier management of cash flow.

All mortgages include covenants. These are the terms that indicate to the borrower the following factors:

- The amount borrowed
- The interest rate being charged, including closing costs, fees, and late charges
- Monthly payment amount and due date of payment
- Past due date and when late charges apply
- Terms of default or foreclosure
- Any collateral pledged toward the debt repayment
- Mortgage holder rights under the terms of the mortgage

Other forms of debt commonly used in buying, building, or operating assisted living communities include the following:

- Leases on buildings and equipment
- Lines of credit for working capital
- Vehicle loans and/or leases
- Vendor carry on **inventories**

Lenders require that there are sufficient funds from operations to cover the debt they are placing on a community. The debt service coverage ratio is a way to quickly determine whether there is adequate cash to cover a loan. A debt coverage ratio of 1.1 or higher indicates that there are sufficient inflows of cash. In corporate finance, it is the amount of cash flow available to meet annual interest and principal payments on debt, including sinking fund payments.

In general, it is calculated by the following formula:

$$\frac{\text{Net Operating Income}}{\text{Total Debt Service}}$$

Contracts

Another area under financing is the development and use of contracts. By definition a contract is an agreement between two or more parties that spells out the obligations of and benefits to each party. It is usually defined in legal language. It outlines the conditions to which all parties must agree.

An assisted living administrator will usually deal with three types of contracts: professional, vendor, and resident. Professional contracts include the type of agreement between other healthcare professionals and the community. Vendor contracts outline agreements with outside service providers. Resident contracts outline the conditions and payments for rent and services between the assisted living community and the resident.

Area of Understanding VI

Maintain appropriate insurance coverage to protect the RC/AL living community.

Insurance provides a way to transfer risk associated with the operation of an RC/AL living community. An RC/AL administrator must aware of the various types of insurance available and how they are used.

Typically, there are five different types of insurance that an administrator will be responsible for managing:

- Property and casualty insurance
- Professional liability insurance
- Auto or vehicle insurance
- Employee health insurance
- Directors and officers insurance (errors and omissions)

Let's take a look at each of these types of insurance and review their use in an assisted living community. When a community is acquired or constructed, the owners generally secure property and casualty insurance.

Property and Casualty Insurance

Property and casualty insurance is insurance that indemnifies a person with an interest in physical property for its loss or the loss of its income-producing abilities. This definition encompasses all lines of insurance written by property and inland marine insurers.

Within this insurance coverage owners generally insure against the breakdown of boilers, machinery, and electrical equipment. Coverage is typically provided on (1) damage to the equipment, (2) expediting expenses, (3) property damage to the property of others, and (4) supplementary payments; and (5) automatic coverage is provided on additional objects. Coverage can be extended to cover consequential losses and loss from interruption of business.

Business interruption insurance is a commercial property form providing coverage for "indirect losses" resulting from property damage, such as loss of business income and extra expenses incurred. It usually includes a time element coverage that pays for loss of earnings when operations are curtailed or suspended because of property loss as a result of an insured peril.

Business personal property, known as "contents," is also found within the area of property insurance. This term actually refers to furniture, fixtures, equipment, machinery, merchandise, materials, and all other personal property owned by the insured and used in the insured's business.

Providers with multiple communities often group their property insurance under a blanket insurance policy. This is a form of property insurance that covers, in a single contract, either multiple types of property at a single location or one or more types of property at multiple locations.

Professional Liability Insurance

Professional liability insurance is insurance coverage to protect against claims alleging that one's negligence or inappropriate action resulted in bodily injury or property damage.

Coverage for insurance is usually issued on either an occurrence or on claims-made basis. An occurrence basis means that liability coverage extends for injuries or damages that occur during the policy term, regardless of when a claim is actually made. A claim made in the current policy year could be charged against a prior policy year. A claims-made policy provides coverage only if a claim is made during the policy period or any applicable extended reporting period. A claim made during the policy period may be charged against a claims-made policy even if the injury or loss occurred many years prior to the policy period. If a claims-made policy has a retroactive date, an occurrence prior to that date is not covered.

Most insurance policies include a deductible of some amount. A deductible eliminates coverage below a certain threshold dollar amount or is expressed as a percentage. A deductible clause requires the insured to bear risk in each and every loss up to the deductible limit. In theory, deductibles reduce the price of insurance by eliminating numerous small claims that are relatively expensive to handle and also decrease moral hazard.

Other key terms about insurance include the following:

- *Effective date.* The date on which coverage is deemed to be effective under the terms of the policy (claims-made or occurrence).
- *Limits of liability "per claim" and limits in the "aggregate."* An insurance policy may contain a specified limit expressed in a dollar value beyond which the insurance policy will not offer coverage for a single claim. Additionally, a professional liability insurance policy may contain an overall aggregate limiting the total value of all claims made during the term of the policy.
- *Self-insured retention ("SIR").* An amount that the insured elects to self-insure prior to the attachment of the limits of a liability insurance policy. An SIR is generally considerably larger than a deductible and may be used to moderate the costs of the purchase of insurance.
- *Tail (Extended reporting period coverage).* In the event an occurrence insurance policy is purchased to replace a claims-made policy, insurance coverage may not be available for a claim arising during the period of claims-made coverage unless the insured has purchased an extended reporting period under the claims-made policy. Purchasing tail coverage may also be advisable when changing insurance brokers.

Auto or Vehicle Insurance

Auto or vehicle insurance is a form of insurance that protects against losses involving autos. Different types are available depending on the needs and wants of those buying policies. Examples of coverage types include bodily injury liability, property damage liability, medical payments, and collision and comprehensive coverage for physical damage to the insured's vehicle.

Employee Health Insurance

Employee health insurance provides coverage against loss by sickness or bodily injury.

The generic form for this type of insurance provides lump sum or periodic payments in the event of loss occasioned by bodily injury, sickness or disease, and medical expense. The term *health insurance* is now used to replace such terms as *accident insurance, sickness insurance, medical expense insurance, accidental death insurance,* and *dismemberment insurance.* The form is sometimes called accident and health, accident and sickness, accident, or disability income insurance.

Directors and Officers Insurance

Directors and officers insurance provides coverage for directors and officers of a company during the course of their work in providing management oversight and policy guidance to the organization. This coverage typically covers any actual or alleged act, error or omission, misstatement, misleading statement, or breach of fiduciary duty or other duty by an insured person in his or her capacity as an insured person. It also typically covers the following items:

- Any employment practices wrongful act by an insured person
- Any securities activity wrongful act
- Any employment practices wrongful act

Area of Understanding VII

Develop and implement a system to periodically monitor and adjust financial performance.

Financial management of an assisted living community requires careful monitoring of many areas of financial performance. This includes everything from collecting the monthly resident rent to paying vendor bills. In developing systems to monitor overall financial performance, it is imperative that the administrator understand the interrelationships of the various control systems within the community. The administrator must be comfortable with how these interlocking control systems are managed by staff and how information flows to financial reporting structures. The level at which these systems are monitored determines the degree of responsiveness that the community provides when change is necessary.

Some of the more important systems that are monitored and rolled up are described in the following subsections.

System 1: Revenue Management

Let's begin with the basics. All residents must be assessed for level of need. Services are delivered by staff. Services are delivered in units of time, and staff members are paid in units of time. This creates a common denominator for use in monitoring performance. Time can be used to determine efficiency and effectiveness as well as to help administrators ensure that quality care is being delivered. This process then drives service delivery, staffing levels, and resident charges. For providers that do not use time as the common denominator for managing and monitoring, the result is generally that systems are disconnected. This often results in poor quality and excessive **cost creep**

(Moore 2004). See Figure 7.1 for more details.

System 2: Purchasing and Expense Management

The second area of monitoring is operating costs. This includes the interconnected systems of budgeting, budget control management, ordering, vendor billing, and payment. All departments within a community should be familiar with their department budgets. Dollars should be allocated to departments from the community master budget based on the community's overall performance. Department heads should track purchases using budget control forms and a purchase order system. Purchase orders should be matched to invoices when received and paid by financial accounting staff based on the cash disbursement schedule of the community. The checks and balances in this system should ensure that all goods are from approved vendors from approved supply lists and that payments are made only following receipt and acknowledgment of the incurred debt. See Figure 7.2 for more details.

Figure 7.1 Flow of revenue management system.

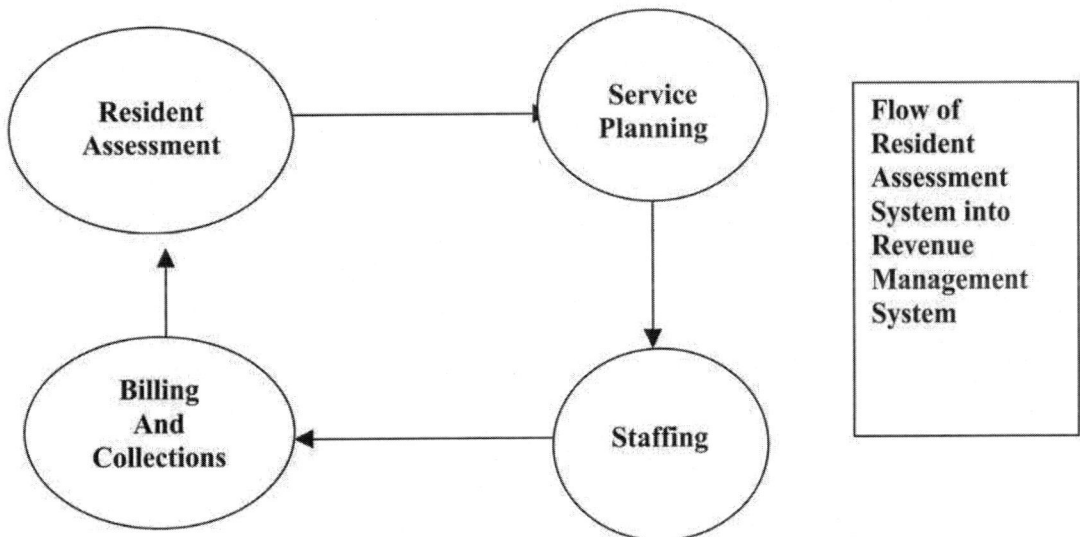

Resident Assessment → Service Planning → Staffing → Billing And Collections → Resident Assessment

Flow of Resident Assessment System into Revenue Management System

Figure 7.2 Flow of purchasing system.

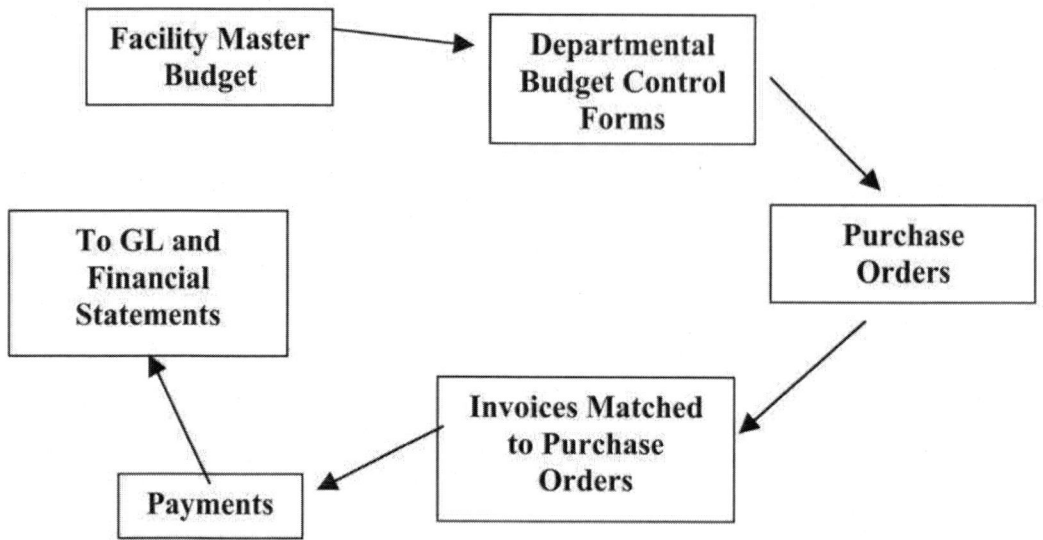

System 3: Financial Performance Management

The third area of monitoring is financial performance management. This includes the review and analysis of monthly and year-to-date financial statements. This generally includes a comparison of actual financial performance to budget. This information is typically examined on a variance basis and may be reviewed in dollars or as a percentage of the budget. This comparison may also look at actual versus budgeted performance on a dollars per resident per day basis.

System 4: Cash Management

The fourth area monitored each month is cash management. This process monitors and reviews the cash inflows and outflows of the community. Revenues collected for rent and services are the primary inflows of cash. As such, accounts receivable must be carefully monitored to ensure that funds are being collected on a timely basis. Outflows include such items as payroll, operating expenses, and financial obligations for things such as mortgages. For communities to remain solvent, they must have adequate working capital to meet these short-term obligations.

System 5: Benchmarking

The concept of benchmarking performance is relatively new to the industry. The National Investment Center (NIC.org) has begun to publish data that allows providers to compare their operating performance against others in the industry. This concept helps providers determine whether their operating results are similar to others. For example: Food cost is typically compared as a dollar per resident day amount. If your community is spending $5.00 per day and others are spending $4.00 per day, you may want to examine where you are spending your money. Communities are typically compared on other items such as occupancy, fill-up rates, and net operating income expressed as a percentage of operating costs divided by revenues. By reviewing this information on a routine basis providers can gain a better understanding of how their systems are functioning compared to others in the industry.

GLOSSARY

Account: A statement summarizing the record of transactions in the form of credits, debits, accruals, and adjustments that have occurred and have an effect on an asset, equity, liability, or past, present, or future revenue.

Account balance: The net of debits and credits for an account at the end of a reporting period. This applies for all types of accounts. A bank account balance shows the amount owed to you by the bank whereas a credit card balance shows the amount you owe to the credit card company.

Accounting period: A specific period of time in which the activities of a company are summarized, usually a year.

Accounts payable: Money owed by a company to those with which it does business. It is also an accounting entry that represents an entity's obligation to pay cash to its creditors. The accounts payable entry is found on a balance sheet under the heading current liabilities. Accounts payable are often referred to as payables. Think of the phone company, the gas company, and the community food vendor as types of creditors. Each demands payment for goods or services rendered and must be paid accordingly. If a community doesn't pay its bills, it is considered to be in default.

Accounts receivable: Money owed by customers (residents or others) to a community in exchange for goods or services that have been delivered or used but not yet paid for. Accounts receivable usually come in the form of operating lines of credit and are usually due within a relatively short time period, ranging from a few days or weeks to a year. Most accounts receivable in assisted living are for services billed in advance.

If you look at the balance sheet of an assisted living community, you will usually see accounts receivable recorded as an asset because they represent a legal obligation for the customer to remit cash for its debts. Accounts receivable are not limited to businesses—individuals have them as well. People get receivables from their employers on a monthly or biweekly basis in the form of a paycheck. They are legally owed this money for services (work) provided.

Accrued interest payable: A current liability account that shows amount of interest accrued on a company debt even though it has not been charged with interest.

Amortization: Process of paying off a liability, deferred charge, or capital expense over some period of time.

Auditing: The process of checking records and reports to make sure they are accurate.

Assets: Property used in operation of the company, that includes cash, buildings, good will, land, and so forth.

Balance sheet: Shows the financial position at any given point in time. This statement gives information about assets, liabilities, and equities of a community.

Breakeven point: Level of operation at which dollars received from sales just cover fixed overhead and the variable costs involved in operations.

Budget: Operating road map of future financial performance. Budgets outline company and individual goals and responsibility and a measure for evaluating performance.

Chart of accounts: An index showing the order and numbering of all the accounts in a ledger.

Control systems: A system designed to manage a specific operating system. A control system for managing departmental purchases might include a beginning monthly budget amount that gets translated to a monthly budget control sheet. Monthly purchase order amounts are then recorded on the sheet showing a remaining balance. As goods are received, purchases are matched to invoices to ensure that the correct goods and prices are received and that payment is made.

Cost accounting: Deals with the measurement and allocation of costs to be assigned to a service or a phase of a service or production.

Cost creep: The increasing of costs (usually labor) as a result of increased resident acuity (need) without any corresponding increase in revenue as an offset.

Current assets: Cash and its equivalents, receivable, inventories.

Current ratio: Current assets divided by current liabilities; determines how financially sound the company is. The wider the margin by which current assets exceeds current liabilities, the sounder the company.

Debit/credit: Credit: An accounting entry system that either decreases assets or increases liabilities. Debit: An accounting entry that results in either an increase in assets or a decrease in liabilities on a company's balance sheet or in your bank account.

Depreciation: System of allocating original cost of an item over the expected life of the item, which is charged off as part of the cost as an expense on each accounting period.

Equities: Rights to the assets. Either (1) creditors; through loans, are debts of business; (2) proprietors; through money invested by people in the company (owners equity).

FICA tax: Social security taxes, FOB Federal Old Age Benefits Tax.

Fiscal year: Yearly accounting period used by a company. Any 12-month period chosen by the company for computing and reporting profits.

Fixed assets: Fairly permanent, used in the business, not bought for resale.

Fixed charges: Interest charges, rent, lease payments, debt payments.

Income statement: Shows revenues, expenses, and net results of a business operation for a given period.

Inventories: Goods on hand, raw material, supplies.

Journal: Primary record of every transaction in chronological order.

Ledger: Group of accounts used by a company.

Liabilities: Debts, ownership by stockholders (payable), reserves, claims against company.

Modeling: A process by which various operational scenarios are tested using a computer-based program to determine the optimal solution for an operational problem.

Net worth: Represents excess of assets over liabilities, also known as stockholder's equity or capital.

Salary: Compensations paid to those at managerial levels.

Time and acuity: Terms used to help providers understand the common elements of operation. Salary and wages are paid based on time just as care is delivered in time increments. Acuity is a means of translating resident care needs into segments of time.

Unearned revenue: Revenue collected in advance or prepaid revenue. Most assisted living communities collect rent in advance. This is then earned throughout the month.

Voucher: A form on which a liability is recorded, in addition to information about how and when the liability is paid.

Wages: Describe sums paid to workers on an hourly or weekly basis.

Working capital: Equal to current liabilities minus current assets plus net income, depreciation, deferred taxes, and proceeds from any sale of noncurrent assets.

PRACTICE QUESTIONS

Read each of the following items carefully, and then select the best response.

1. The Civil Rights Act of 1964 in the United States outlaws discrimination based on:
   A. race, color, religion, sex, or national origin.
   B. race, color, religion, sex, or marital status.
   C. race, color, state of residence, sex, or marital status.
   D. race, state of residence, religion, sex, or national origin.

   A B C D
   ○ ○ ○ ○

2. The act which requires the establishment of national standards for electronic healthcare transactions and identifiers for health insurance plans is known as:
   A. FMLA
   B. OSHA
   C. COBRA
   D. HIPPA

   A B C D
   ○ ○ ○ ○

3. The balance sheet is a financial statement that summarizes which of the following items for a for-profit company?
   A. Assets, liabilities, and shareholders' equity at a point in time
   B. Income and expenses for the month or for the year
   C. Change in financial position fur the current period
   D. Legal liabilities and future business obligations

   A B C D
   ○ ○ ○ ○

4. To accurately forecast revenues, an administrator must understand which of the following items?
   A. Current market conditions
   B. Census patterns and trends
   C. Resident acuity and turnover
   D. All of the above

   A B C D
   ○ ○ ○ ○

5. Which financial document contains cash flows from operating, investing, and financing activities; as well as acts as kind of corporate checkbook?
   A. Chart of Accounts
   B. Balance Sheet
   C. Income Statement
   D. Cash Flow Statement

   A B C D
   ○ ○ ○ ○

6. Net profit margin is:
   A. Net Income + Interest Expense divided by Total Assets
   B. EBITDA divided by Interest Expense
   C. Net Income divided by Revenue
   D. Service Revenue divided by Service Cost

   A B C D
   ○ ○ ○ ○

7. Working Capital Ratio is:
   A. Cash + Accounts Receivable + Short-term Investments divided by Current Liabilities
   B. Current Assets divided by Current Liabilities
   C. Accounts Receivable divided by (Revenue / 365)
   D. Total Liabilities divided by Total Assets

   A B C D
   ○ ○ ○ ○

8. An example of a variable cost is the:
   A. administrator's salary.
   B. mortgage payment.
   C. property taxes.
   D. laundry expenses.

   A B C D
   ○ ○ ○ ○

9. Directors and officers insurance provide coverage for all of the following *except* a/an:
   A. actual or alleged act.
   B. error or omission.
   C. misleading statement.
   D. damage to property.

   A B C D
   ○ ○ ○ ○

10. Assessment system monitoring ties together which of the following subsystems?
    A. Assessment—Services—Staffing—Billing—Purchase Order
    B. Assessment—Services—Contracts—Billing—Payment
    C. Assessment—Services—Staffing—Billing—Collections
    D. Assessment—Budget Control—Staffing—Billing—Collections

    A B C D
    ○ ○ ○ ○

ANSWERS AND EXPLANATIONS

1. **Correct answer = A.** Title VII of the act outlaws discrimination in employment in any business on the basis of race, color, religion, sex, or national origin. Although each of the answers has pieces of the correct response, only answer A lists all four areas of discrimination.

2. **Correct answer = D.** Title II of HIPAA, the Administrative Simplification provisions, requires the establishment of national standards for electronic healthcare transactions and national identifiers for providers, health insurance plans, and employers.

3. **Correct answer = A.** In the for-profit arena, the balance sheet is the financial statement that summarizes a company's assets, liabilities, and shareholders' equity at a specific point in time. The three balance sheet segments give owners, investors, and other stakeholders a summary of what the company owns and owes, as well as the amount invested by the shareholders. The best answer is A. This talks about the three parts of the balance sheet. Answer B refers to the income statement and not the balance sheet. Answer C references the cash flow statement, and answer D references only part of the balance sheet.

4. **Correct answer = D.** To forecast revenues the administrator must understand a number of important areas. These include current market conditions, census patterns and trends, and acuity and turnover. The best answer is D, all of the above.

5. **Correct answer = D.** The cash flow statement generally shows cash flows in and out of the organization in three areas. These include cash flow from operating activities, cash flows from investing activities, and cash flows from financing activities. Whereas the balance sheet gives a one-time snapshot of a company's assets and liabilities and the income statement indicates the business's profitability during a certain period, the cash flow statement acts as a kind of corporate checkbook that reconciles the other two statements.

6. **Correct answer = C.** Profit margin is defined as the ratio of income to sales. There are two types of profit margin: gross profit margin and net profit margin. Gross profit margin shows the percentage return that the facility is earning over the cost of providing services. It is defined as gross profit divided by sales. Net profit shows the percentage of net income generated by each service in for-profit facilities. It is defined as net income divided by sales.

7. **Correct answer = B.** This ratio indicates if a firm has enough short-term assets to cover its immediate liabilities. If the ratio is less than 1, the firm has negative working capital. Caution: Even if current ratio is adequately calculated for the year, there may be periods within the year when there is inadequate cash to pay bills. This is defined as current assets divided by current liabilities.

8. **Correct answer = D.** Typically, there are five different types of insurance that an administrator will be responsible for managing. They include property and casualty insurance, professional liability insurance, auto or vehicle insurance, employee health insurance, and directors and officers insurance (errors and omissions). Answers A, B, and C each lists a portion of the answer; answer D is the best answer because it covers all of the correct elements listed in answers A–C.

9. **Correct answer = D.** This insurance provides coverage for directors and officers of a company during the course of their work in providing management oversight and policy guidance to the organization. This coverage typically covers any actual or alleged act, error or omission, misstatement, misleading statement, or breach of fiduciary duty or other

duty by an insured person in his or her capacity as an insured person. It also typically covers (1) any employment practices wrongful act by an insured person, (2) any securities activity wrongful act, and (3) any employment practices wrongful act.

10. **Correct answer = C.** All residents must be assessed for level of need. Services are delivered by staff. Services are delivered in units of time, and staff members are paid in units of time. This creates a common denominator for use in monitoring performance. Time can be used to determine efficiency and effectiveness as well as to help administrators ensure that quality care is being delivered. This process then drives service delivery, staffing levels, and resident charges. For providers that do not use time as the common denominator for managing and monitoring, the result is generally that systems are disconnected. This often results in poor quality and excessive cost creep.

REFERENCES

Allen, J. 2005. *Assisted Living Administration*. 2nd ed. New York: Springer Publishing Company.

American Association of Homes and Services for the Aging (AAHSA). 1995. *Operational Practices in Assisted Living/Residential Care—AAHSA's Wellness Model*. Washington, DC: AAHSA.

American Association of Homes and Services for the Aging (AAHSA). 1996a. *Assisted Living Underwriting Guidelines*. Washington, DC: AAHSA.

American Association of Homes and Services for the Aging (AAHSA). 1996b. *Financial Ratios and Trends Analyses*. Washington, DC: AAHSA.

American Health Care Association (AHCA). 1997. *Satisfaction Assessment Questionnaire for Assisted Residents*. Washington, DC: AHCA.

Anderson, J.R. 1996. *Budgeting and Purchasing Capital Equipment*. Washington, DC: AAHSA.

Assisted Living Federation of America (ALFA). 1997. *Orientation to Assisted Living*. Oakton, VA: ALFA.

Brown, S., and A. Bass. 1990. *Americans with Disabilities Act of 1990: A Guide to Compliance*. New York: West Publishing.

Coopers & Lybrand L.L.P. 1996. *Overview of the Assisted Living Industry*. Fairfax, VA: Assisted Living Federation of America.

Drucker, P.F. 1993. *Management: Tasks, Responsibilities, Practices*. New York: Harper Business Publishing.

Goldsmith, S.B. .1993. *Long Term Care Administrator's Handbook*. New York: Aspen Publishing.

Hawkins, R.W. 2004. *Management Accounting for Health Care Organizations: Tools and Techniques for Decision Support*. Sudbury, MA: Jones and Bartlett.

Ittelson, T. 1998. *Financial Statements: A Step-by-Step Guide to Understanding and Creating Financial Reports*. Franklin Lakes, NJ: Career Press.

Kane, R.A., and K. Brown Wilson. 1993. *Assisted Living in the United States. A New Paradigm for Residential Care for Frail Older Persons?* Washington, DC: American Association of Retired Persons.

Moore, J. 1996. *Assisted Living, Pure and Simple Development and Operating Strategies*. Fort Worth, TX: Westridge Publishing.

National Center for Assisted Living (NCAL). 2005. *Facts and Trends—the Assisted Living Source Book*. Fairfax, VA: NCAL.

Occupational Safety and Health Administration. 1997. *OSHA Recordkeeping*. Chap. 1710. Washington, DC: Bureau of National Affairs.

Roush, D.A., and T.H. Grape. 1996. *Integrated Senior Care: Assisted Living and Long-Term Care Manual*. New York: Thompson Publishing Group.

Smith, B., and E. Wiening. 1994. *How Insurance Works*. 2nd ed. Malvern, PA: Insurance Institute of America.

U.S. Department of Labor. 1997. *OSHA Handbook for Small Business*. Washington, DC: U.S. Department of Labor.

APPENDIX 7.A

Popular methods of evaluating capital budget items include net present value (NPV), internal rate of return (IRR), discounted cash flow (DCF), and payback period.

NPV

The difference between the present value of cash inflows and the present value of cash outflows. NPV is used in capital budgeting to analyze the profitability of an investment or project.

NPVvanalysis is sensitive to the reliability of future cash inflows that an investment or project will yield.

Formula:

$$NPV = \sum_{t=1}^{T} \frac{C_t}{(1 + r)^t} - C_0$$

NPV compares the value of a dollar today to the value of that same dollar in the future, taking inflation and returns into account. If the NPV of a prospective project is positive, it should be accepted. However, if NPV is negative, the project should probably be rejected because cash flows will also be negative.

IRR

Often used in capital budgeting, IRR is the interest rate that makes net present value of all cash flow equal zero.

Essentially, this is the return that a company would earn if it expanded or invested in itself, rather than investing that money elsewhere.

DCF

A valuation method used to estimate the attractiveness of an investment opportunity. Discounted cash flow (DCF) analysis uses future free cash flow projections and discounts them (most often using the weighted average cost of capital) to arrive at a present value, which is used to evaluate the potential for investment. If the value arrived at through DCF analysis is higher than the current cost of the investment, the opportunity may be a good one.

DCF is calculated as:

$$DCF = \frac{CF_1}{(1 + r)^1} + \frac{CF_2}{(1 + r)^2}$$
$$+ \cdots + \frac{CF_n}{(1 + r)^n}$$

$$CF = \text{Cash Flow}$$
$$r = \text{discount rate (WACC)}$$

CHAPTER 8

PERSON-CENTERED CARE IN ASSISTED LIVING

Karen Love, Pathways to Care and Mauro Hernandez, Concepts for Community Living

Introduction

While the Second Edition of the *Residential Care/Assisted Living Administrators Exam Study Guide* incorporates aspects of person-centered care in its curriculum, this chapter expands on the requisite knowledge. An understanding of person-centered care is imperative for today's residential care/assisted living administrators as this approach is becoming more and more recognized as the gold standard.

Over the past 20 years or so, much has been written about both assisted living and person-centered care. Person-centered care has become a dominant approach in various models to improve quality of care and life embraced by consumers, regulators, advocates, and, in many cases, providers. Interestingly, although not often explicitly recognized, the principles of person-centered care are viewed by many providers as inherent in the widely recognized and adopted principles of assisted living. As noted further below, these include the values of individuality, choice, privacy, dignity, independence, and a home environment in which to reside. Proponents of the Pioneer Network hold a broader view of person-centered care to include evidence-based practices for: relationships and community; governance; leadership; services; engagement; specialized skills such as dementia care; and accountability.

This chapter begins by reviewing the origins of assisted living and its early conceptualization of person-centered care followed by a wider examination of it.

Origins of Assisted Living

The early predecessors to purpose-built assisted livings included small "family-style" board and care homes that provided personal care, shelter and oversight to a handful of clients (Pratt, 2004). Larger "homes for the aged" have been around since at least the late 1800s and were often owned and operated by state or county governments to meet the housing and care needs of poor older citizens. More recent forms of long-term residential care have included campus style communities, smaller adult foster homes, and larger adult group housing settings with coordinated services (Kane & Wilson, 1993). Labeled by different names, such as boarding homes and residential care facilities, supply for these types of facilities continued to grow modestly and with limited public attention well into the 1980s.

During the late 1980's and early 1990's, the term "assisted living" emerged to describe a newer model of residential care—distinct from what is known as "board and care." Assisted living grew rapidly as a result of market response to changing consumer preferences, the growing availability of development capital, and shifts in state long-term care policies (Hawes et al, 1999; Wilson, 1995). Innovators on both coasts (Klaassen and Wilson) were designing this new residential care setting to blend elements found in traditional homes with a more enhanced service capacity than found in traditional board and care (Wilson, 2007).

State fiscal concerns and consumer advocacy efforts led states to expand the supply of and access to nursing home alternatives. Assisted living was viewed as one of several options that could reduce nursing home use and associated Medicaid costs by either diverting or delaying nursing home placement (J. Wiener & D. G. Stevenson, 1998). Additionally, a growing number of older consumers had more disposable income and greater assets than in previous decades.

Aspects of Person-Centered Care as a Core Concept in Assisted Living

Early conceptualization about assisted living as a distinct service delivery model represented a response to a number of concerns with existing long-term care options that were recognized as being overly medicalized, institutional and impersonal. A set of core values was theorized for assisted living based on specific and interconnected philosophical, environmental, and programmatic components that would be more responsive to consumer needs and preferences than traditional residential care settings.

The early concepts of assisted living are important to understand as they laid the foundation for aspects of person-centered care in assisted living and other settings. One foundational component was that the physical environment should be designed to be more like "home" in terms of scale and architectural style (Wilson, 2007). Universal design approaches were incorporated to accommodate changing needs. Individual living spaces in assisted living residences included a kitchenette for food preparation and storage, a private full bathroom with a roll-in shower, and a lockable front door—a significant

departure from shared living spaces in nursing homes.

Second, a more comprehensive, flexible, and less medically oriented package of services was emphasized that would enable residents to play a more active role in meeting their own needs and preferences (Wilson, 1995). Table 1 provides detail about this component. The third major component was an overarching philosophical orientation that infused the environment and services with values such as privacy, individuality, choice, dignity, independence, and a residential environment. Principles of individuality and choice require services to be tailored to each individual's unique preferences and circumstances. This personalization is reflected in a plan of services negotiated with the resident (and/or her representative) that specifies how and when services are to be provided. The values of individuality and choice view each resident as the center of decision-making involving their lives. As opposed to being an "object of care," the individual's preferences are central in the selection and organization of services. Although dignity can be a more amorphous term, in assisted living it has been defined as a term to convey the fundamental right of individuals living in licensed residential settings to be listened to, as well as to be treated with respect, courtesy, and in age appropriate ways.

Diverging Concepts of Person-Centered Care

The early assisted living pioneers of the late 1980s began using the term "resident-centered care" to describe the above referenced collective changes they were implementing in this newly forming industry. At approximately the same time, the U.S. Congress legislated sweeping changes for certified nursing homes (the Omnibus Budget Reconciliation Act (OBRA) of 1987) that mandated a national minimum set of standards of care and rights. A significant aspect of the changes

Table 1. Key Constructs in Assisted Living	
Concept	**Specification**
Normalized environments and homelike residential features	a. Architectural style commonly associated with places people have lived and that is thematically recognizable as residential (e.g., with building materials, design, and furnishings found in private homes).
	b. Interior community space to accommodate recognized public functions (e.g., dining, socializing, shopping, receiving services).
	c. Accommodation of cultural preferences for privacy (e.g., control over entry to and use of one's personal living space, provisions for bathing and toilet use and for storing and preparing food in one's personal space, no requirements to share personal living space with others unless by choice).
	d. Amenities in public and in personal space consistent with encouraging choice and continuity of life experiences (e.g., amount and type of community space, size of personal living space, temperature in personal living space).
	e. Scale (size) and setting (location) congruent with older adults' life experiences in their own communities (e.g., rural, small town, suburban, or urban communities; different cultural communities).
	f. Feature to accommodate the individual's changing abilities (e.g., universal design features such as adjustable closets, level door hardware; 100% wheelchair-accessible units and common space; roll-in showers to facilitate the ability to remain in the setting if the tenant chooses).
Enhanced service capacity to foster residents' well-being	a. Ability to provide assistance with activities of daily living and instrumental activities of daily living when needed and wanted (e.g., capacity to meet scheduled and unscheduled needs at a time agreed to by the consumer by a universal worker trained to accommodate most needs).
	b. Appropriate interventions to manage the effects of chronic disease or disability (e.g., the ability to provide health-related services associated with assessment of condition; plan negotiated with the consumer and/or the family for needed services, management of medication use, direct or delegated nursing treatments; follow-through with ordered therapies; and end-of-life palliative care).

continued

Table 1. Key Constructs in Assisted Living *continued*	
Concept	**Specification**
	c. Arrangement for treatment of acute care episodes and mental health issues (e.g., identification, coordination, and monitoring of condition to ensure timely intervention in the assisted living community or by transfer to another setting for specialized treatments; hospital, psychiatric unit, skilled nursing facility, rehabilitation center).
	d. Attention to all aspects of well-being (e.g., emotional support of individual tenant and his or her family, opportunities to form new relationships and to engage in activities of personal interest, opportunities to be spiritual in a way acceptable to the individual, opportunities to experience continued personal growth).
	e. Responsibility for the coordination (case management) of services needed for enhanced well-being (e.g., arrangement of services of any type not specifically available in the assisted living community, oversight of transitional events such as move in and move out).
Values orientation to preserve residents' self-worth	a. A focus on ability as opposed to disability (e.g., to support the highest level of independence possible to meeting self-needs and to assist in motivating individuals to set personal goals for increased ability for self-care).
	b. Focus on decision making, both decisional and executional autonomy (e.g., to offer choices in a way that encourages, facilitates, and respects decisions at all levels of importance.
	c. Focus on personalization (e.g., to recognize the uniqueness of each individual and to capture that individuality in a negotiated service agreement in partnership with the consumer and his or her family).
	d. Focus on reciprocity (e.g., to recognize and promote mutual respect, dignity, and responsibility to be shared by the consumer, the caregiver, and those of special importance to the consumer, such as the family).
	e. Focus on boundaries (e.g., to uphold the personal boundaries related to privacy involving emotional intimacy, information, and the physical body; to use techniques like managed risk agreements as a means to identify and establish boundaries around decision and subsequent behaviors that might cause harm to the person).

Source: Wilson 2007

included an emphasis on a resident's quality of life as well as the quality of care (Turnham). A national effort among proponents of OBRA began to take shape across the country to transform the culture and environments in institutional long-term care to homey, life-affirming settings in which elders self-direct their care and are treated with respect and dignity. These transformers of change began using the term "person-centered care."

Both groups used the related terms to refer to changes in the physical environment (homey), service delivery (resident-directed), and core values (dignity, respect, choice, and privacy). As abundant research efforts began providing advances to improve practices, the term person-centered care began to refer to a widening set of core components that were not necessarily also being adopted by assisted living. As the ranks of the nursing home proponents swelled, this transformative movement, known informally as the culture change movement, was formalized in the early 1990's through the creation of a nonprofit organization—the Pioneer Network. The Pioneer Network broadened its purview in the late 2000s from nursing homes to include all long-term care settings including assisted living, adult day services and home care, and is the leading national proponent of person-centered care in LTC.

Person-Centered Care—National Background

Some entities and organizations use terms other than person-centered care including: patient-centered care; person-centered thinking, resident-centered care, resident-directed care; and patient-directed care. The variety of terms used reflect word distinctions in two areas. One variance is the use of the term 'person' over 'resident' or 'patient.' Many prefer the use of 'person' as being a more holistic term that incorporates the whole care network as well as the elder. The other variance is between the terms 'centered' and 'directed' with some preferring 'directed' as better describing elders' choice and control values while others feel that 'centered' encompasses the broader realm such as for those with dementia that may no longer be able to 'direct' their care. The best term yet may be the one that Planetree Alliance is beginning to use—relationship-centered care as it may best denote the importance of relationships. The term 'person-centered care' is used here because it is the more widely used term in the aging literature (Bowers, 2009).

Tom Kitwood, a British gerontologist, was one of the first to use the term "person-centered care" in the field of aging to describe an empowering philosophy of care that rebalances work priorities from a focus on accomplishing tasks to a focus on the person needing assistance (Fazio, 2008). Care is not organized for staff convenience, efficiency or other such criteria. Person-centered care proponents view institutional long-term care as having been primarily task-orientated both for efficiency reasons and due to the prevalence of hierarchical management systems. The Eden Alternative® is one of the first nationally organized efforts to implement person-centered care in nursing homes. It codifies the need to rebalance the nexus of decision-making to the elder or as close to them as possible ensuring that they direct their own daily schedules and preferences among other needs (Lustbader & Williams, 2006).

There are a number of other organized national efforts underway to implement person-centered care in hospitals, nursing homes, and assisted living. Planetree, founded in 1978, dedicated itself to radically changing the way health care was delivered in hospitals (Frampton, Gilpin & Charmel, 2003). Planetree has since broadened its purview to include the wider spectrum of care settings including long-term care. Other organized national transformative efforts include the Wellspring Program, GREEN HOUSES®, the Household Model, and Dementia Care Mapping [see Resources at the end of this chapter for information to learn more about these efforts]. The common goal among them is to realign operational practices to provide person-centered care thus enhancing the care and service recipients' experience. Some of these efforts are very specific and prescriptive such as Green Houses® while others simply set forth a set of core principles.

The Green House®/assisted living are referenced in the chapter as it is the only nationally recognized model of care in assisted living that fully incorporate all aspects of person-centered care. The Green House®/assisted living model sets specific guidelines such as community size, interior design features, and staffing roles and responsibilities among others. The primary purpose of Green Houses®/ assisted living are to create a home in which elders can thrive. Elders receive assistance and services without the assistance and services becoming the focus of their lives. At the core of the Green House®/assisted living culture are relationships; relationships among and between staff, residents, families and friends. Development of Green Houses®/ assisted living communities are only considered in states that have regulations that support 'aging in place.'

Person-centered care has become almost trendy, some viewing it as a "litmus test for being politically correct" (Smull, 2000). To actually achieve person-centered care, however, requires deep systems and organizational changes that reflect different values, beliefs and practices at all levels including what constitutes: good care; a good environment in which to live; and a good environment in which to work. These efforts, however, are yielding dramatically positive results for residents, their families and the staff caring for them (Kantor, et al, 2009).

Studies to date have mostly focused on selected aspects of person-centered care, which may provide a confusing and incomplete landscape of person-centered care. There are no known publications that examine all the components and evidence-based practices of person-centered care. The Pioneer Network and the Center for Excellence in Assisted Living (CEAL) have prepared papers to more clearly define person-centered care and identify the key structural elements that are needed to support it in the nursing home and assisted living settings respectively. This chapter provides a holistic framework of person-centered care concepts, structures and practices that are applicable to assisted living based on a comprehensive review of the literature, as well as interviews and discussions with person-centered care experts in the aging services field.

What is Person-Centered Care

While there is as yet no common agreement about what constitutes quality or how it should be measured in assisted living, there is strong consensus that optimizing resident well-being is a desired outcome (Zimmerman et al, 2008). Person-centered care focuses both on quality of life and quality of care with the goal of optimizing resident well-being. Relationships among staff, residents and families are at the heart of person-centered care. It is a transformation from a paternalistic/ maternalistic model of care to a consumer-directed model that honors elders' life experiences, interests, routines of daily life through relationships.

The elements needed to support person-centered care for nursing home residents and individuals with developmental disabilities have been more widely studied and published. To our knowledge, there has been no research conducted about person-centered care in assisted living. GREEN HOUSES® licensed as assisted living and anecdotal evidence are providing information that the structural elements needed to support person-centered care in assisted living are very similar to those in nursing homes. Since there is little assisted living-specific person-centered care research available, research conducted in other settings such as nursing homes, as appropriate, are cited.

Person-centered care's foundation is based on the traditional assisted living values noted above, as well as a philosophy of relationship-based care and services that optimizes resident well-being. The work culture realigns priorities, structures and processes to best support conditions conducive to normal life with a focus on residents' preferences, routines, and needs rather than residents following the care setting's routines or schedules (Fazio, 2008). These outcomes are achieved by implementing a new work culture. The term 'culture' is carefully selected and important because it denotes the totality of organizational structure. Besides the core values and philosophy of relationship-based care and services, the totality of organizational structural elements needed to support a culture of person-centered care in assisted living are:

- person-centered care governance
- person-centered care leadership
- person-centered care workforce practices
- person-centered care services
- person-centered environment and design, and
- person-centered engagement

The term 'person-centered care' is used as a qualifier to distinguish each element from other types of leadership, workforce practices, etc. Person-centered care is not a method or set of methods but rather a total reorganization and realignment of systems, structures and processes that transforms traditional staff roles. In order to achieve a culture of person-centered care, an organization has to align and effect all seven elements as well as the values and relationship-based philosophy. Although a focus on implementing one or two elements such as leadership and workforce practices may strengthen operational performance, proponents assert that it does not yield a person-centered care culture.

Person-Centered Care and the NAB Domains

The Second Edition of the *Residential Care/Assisted Living Administrators Exam Study Guide* outlines five domains of practice that are listed below with the corresponding seven person-centered care elements:

Person-Centered Care Values and Relationship-Based Philosophy

The values (respect, autonomy [self-direction and control]; dignity, choice, independence, and privacy) and relationship-based philosophy are the foundation of person-centered care. This personalization upends traditional service delivery that may integrate aspects of customer service (e.g., respect, choice, privacy), and redefines the entire service delivery system. Instead of residents being 'objects of care' that revolve around an organizational structure, the organizational structure revolves around the residents by optimizing respect and courtesy for them and supporting their autonomy, dignity, choice, independence, and privacy.

Person-Centered Care Relationship-Based Philosophy

Positive relationships offer context and meaning to daily life including a sense of belonging. This positive outcome is important not only for the well-being of assisted living residents but also for the staff. "It is through their relationships with residents that staff find meaning in these...jobs. For most (staff), their relationships with residents are the primary component of job satisfaction (Ball et

NAB Domain	PCC Structural Element
Client/Resident Services Management	PCC Services
	PCC Engagement
Human Resources Management	PCC Workforce Practices
Leadership And Governance	PCC Governance
	PCC Leadership
Physical Environment Management	PCC Environment and Design

Note* The following details the person-centered care elements within each NAB domain. This information is not intended as an exhaustive detailing about person-centered care, but rather a solid overview. Additional resource materials are referenced at the end of the chapter for further reading.

al., 2009)." The power and value of relationships can not be overstated. Relationships not only optimize overall resident well-being, but also staff job fulfillment and satisfaction.

Assisted living communities with a culture of person-centered care recognize the importance of committing to an investment in staff time (including staffing workload) in order for relationships to flourish among staff, the residents, family members and others such as volunteers. As with all cultural aspects, new people coming into the community (e.g., residents, staff, families) are oriented to person-centered care's relationship-based philosophy. Many person-centered care communities have a tradition of holding weekly community gatherings using the learning circle technique. The community gathering provides an established mechanism to include all community members in a regular discussion and can be a helpful means for new members to become acquainted with the other community members.

Generally the gatherings are an opportunity to come together and talk but they can also be used to make decisions affecting the assisted living community. The learning circle technique is simple beginning with the 'gathering' of chairs so everyone can sit in a circle. Gatherings have a facilitator who can change each time or rotate among a handful of people. The facilitator poses a question or initiates a point of discussion. Anyone sitting in the circle can decide to speak first with each successive speaker going clockwise or counterclockwise from the first speaker around the circle until everyone has a chance to speak. An individual can 'pass' their turn and opt to speak after everyone has spoken.

Examples of Person-Centered Care Relationship-Based Philosophy

- Staff regularly eat meals with the residents. Mealtime is an interpersonal opportunity to connect and converse with residents and vice versa.
- The assisted living residence has a tradition in how its community members welcome new members.

- The assisted living residence has a tradition in how its community members acknowledge the death of a resident.

Person-Centered Care and NAB's Domain for Leadership and Governance

NAB Definition—Leaders of residential care/assisted living organizations are key in setting the agenda and strategic direction of the organization, managing and motivating personnel, providing critical community connections and relationships, managing problems, and ensuring that systems are in place to achieve quality outcomes.

Person-Centered Care Governance

Governance is the primary and most essential structural element for achieving person-centered care. This is because the culture of an organization is ultimately driven by the organization's highest authority(ies). An enthused leader or charismatic employee may be able to initiate some aspects of person-centered care, but without the commitment and active involvement of the governing authority(ies) sustaining a culture of person-centered care is not achievable. Transformation to a culture of person-centered care should be deeply imbedded in all aspects of an organization including its mission, vision and values statements.

Reported Examples of Governance to Support Person-Centered Care—

- Governing authority(ies) actively are involved in transformational and training activities.
- Governing authority(ies) ensure that the staff have the resources needed to implement and sustain a culture of person-centered care.

Person-Centered Care Leadership

Person-centered care ushers in a transformed organizational chart structure. Rather than a hierarchical diagram of staff responsibilities, it calls for a circular organizational diagram. Person-centered care leaders focus on people; inspire trust; maintain a long range perspective; and are willing to be changed by the ideas and perspectives of others (Kantor et al. (2009). This inspirational leadership style is essential for person-centered care. Research has shown that an autocratic, hierarchical style of leadership is not conducive to person-centered care (Donoghue & Castle, 2009; Holleran, 2007). While there are many models of effective leadership styles, no one style is considered as best suited for person-centered care. All effective leadership styles, however, encompass the following:

- Investing in staff by fostering a continual learning environment both informally (through stand-up meetings and coaching) and formally (through professional trainings, in-services and other educational opportunities).
- Continually recognizing and appreciating staff work efforts through genuine praise and encouragement.
- Modeling effective practices which can motivate and inspire staff.
- Promoting creativity, innovation and problem-solving.
- Allowing staff to make mistakes from which they can learn and also become more empowered and engaged.

Decentralized decision making is an essential leadership practice to support person-centered care (Donoghue and Castle, 2009; Kiefer et al, 2005). Decentralized decision-making occurs when leaders empower staff to address and make decisions and judgments related to their work responsibilities instead of bringing all issues back for leaders to resolve. This leadership style better involves and invests staff in the outcomes of their work efforts, as well as utilizes their increased knowledge of the situation to enhance problem solving techniques. Staff is held accountable for the outcomes generated by their decisions which can provide a useful context in which to help staff learn from mistakes. Decentralized decision-making recognizes that staff have the most knowledge about residents' needs and preferences and as such are in the best position to support residents' interests and needs, and extends to all staff including dining room staff and housekeepers among others.

Reported Examples of Leadership to Support Person-Centered Care—

- Ensuring all staff has opportunities for education, training, skill building, and coaching about person-centered care (See Resource section).
- Maintaining an open communication culture.
- Recognizing and celebrates incremental successes.

Person-Centered Care and NAB's Domain for Human Resources Management

NAB Definition—the effective and efficient management of the people we employ in residential care/assisted living.

Person-Centered Care Workforce Practices

Person-centered care depends on a stable, trained workforce in which everyone (including owners, boards of directors, and corporate executives) is oriented, trained and continually supported in person-centered care techniques. In other words, the entire organizational culture is oriented to the principles and practices of person-centered care. The Better Jobs Better Care national workforce initiative, among other research efforts, has provided

143

valuable and abundant information about workforce practices that can support person-centered care including:

- An organizational culture that values, respects and nurtures all staff;
- Effective staff recruitment and retention practices;
- Appropriately trained staff;
- Appropriate number of staff;
- Effective staff orientation, training, and mentoring for building person-centered care skills and competencies;
- Consistent staffing assignments;
- Self-managed work teams;
- Open, effective communication; and
- Effective managers and supervisors.

Staff satisfaction surveys and research provide evidence that job satisfaction is a key predictor of job stability; the less satisfied, the more likely staff is to leave (Donoghue & Castle, 2009; Barry et al, 2005; Castle & Enberg, 2005; Kemp et al, 2009; Sikorska-Simmons, 2005). A community with high staff turnover has less opportunity for training, supervision, mentoring, and forming and nurturing resident relationships, which in turn result in negative outcomes. Staff instability is not compatible with sustaining person-centered care.

Studies show that the estimated staff turnover cost for each direct care worker is approximately $2,500 (Ferrell & Dawson, 2007; Seavey, 2004)). This amount only includes the direct costs associated with recruiting and training new staff. One report estimated that in a typical assisted living residence with 67 staff and an average turnover rate of 73%, the annual cost associated with new hires was approximately $84,537 (Jacob, 2002).

Staff is frequently placed in situations that require unusually sophisticated interpersonal and communication skills. They are called upon to manage conflict, set limits, make ethical decisions, grieve and help others grieve, and support other members of their team. There is little in staff training that addresses

such complex psychosocial needs (Better Jobs Better Care report No. 3, 2005). For staff to be successful navigating the complex skills required for their jobs, they need to be supported through continuous quality training, coaching and mentoring. Empowering staff to maximize use of their skills and to be provided adequate training and support has been found to minimize stress, reduce turnover and improve care (Hyde et al, 2008).

Traditional teaching methods that rely heavily on lecture and video are not the best learning format (PHI & IFAS, 2005). Interactive and experiential training methods have been found to be more productive and beneficial. This is partly because people have different learning strengths; some learn best visually, others by hearing information and still others by doing. The more participatory and interactive the training, the more likely staff will integrate new knowledge into their understanding and be able to use this new information in their work.

Consistent staffing is another key workforce practice of person-centered care for several reasons. First, staff are better able to become familiar with the residents' typical behaviors, moods, and appearance while also developing the relationship context of person-centered care. Using the example of a resident who prefers a warm evening shower and a cup of tea before bedtime, a consistent staff member not only would know the importance of the evening shower and cup of tea, but also that this is the time of day that this resident likes to sit and talk for five undistracted minutes. This talk time for the resident might represent one of the ways in which she or he feels emotionally connected and nurtured. While spending time talking does not require a large time commitment or highly developed communication skills, it could represent one way that resident feels a sense of belonging in her or his assisted living residence impacting positively upon their emotional well-being.

Staff members that are good at their job are often considered for promotion to supervisory or managerial positions. These positions require a special skill set that staff may not innately have or been trained for, such as critical thinking skills and how to effectively manage people. In order for them to be successful in the new position, a culture of person-centered care ensures that staff are provided with educational opportunities needed to impart the knowledge and skills related to the supervisory or managerial responsibilities that they now have.

Person-centered care maximizes staff empowerment through the formation of self-managed work teams. These are semi-autonomous groups of staff that are empowered and responsible for organizing, decision-making and controlling different aspects of their work. In larger communities, work teams are configured geographically within the assisted living residence to provide care and services for residents living in a neighborhood or one area. The size of the assisted living residence will dictate the number of work teams and the number of members in each work team. The self-managed work teams may consist of several direct care staff and a housekeeper. They take on responsibility including problem-solving, but are accountable for outcomes. Work teams typically have a lead member who is responsible for communicating information to and from others outside their work team. Work teams are cross-trained to be able to help residents with a wide assortment of needs such as laundry, eating a late meal, bathing, light housekeeping, etc.

To help ensure the workforce practices are effective, person-centered care depends upon clear and consistent means of communication among all staff. Because assisted living residence operates 24 hours a day seven days a week, it is impossible to see and talk with all staff on a daily basis. Because person-centered care is based on relationships, regularly gathering staff together in person is important to nurture community among staff. Staff should be encouraged to bring up items for discussion and provide constructive feedback.

It likely will take some trial and error until all staff are effectively communicating together.

Table 2 (see pg. 146) distinguishes key differences between workforce practices and selected outcomes in person-centered care cultures and those of a traditional long-term care culture.

Reported Examples of Human Resources Management to Support Person-Centered Care—

- Staff recognizing and valuing each others successes and contributions.
- Staff holding quarterly pot lucks in order to have interpersonal time together.
- Organization having a welcoming tradition for new staff that includes dining service preparing a special meal that all staff members enjoy with the new staff member.
- Ensuring that new staff member orientation and mentoring programs are taken seriously by all staff to ensure the success of their newest member.
- Teaching managers and supervisors conflict resolution and communication skills to enhance their mentoring and coaching roles.
- Providing education and training to all staff about customer service, problem-solving techniques and root cause analysis.

Person-Centered Care and NAB's Domain for Client/Resident Services Management

NAB Definition—A key concept in resident services provision in residential care/assisted living is person-centered care. The way care is provided and how the resident wants to be cared for serve as direct reflections of the assisted living philosophy in action and ensure that the resident has control of his or her life.

Table 2.	
Person-Centered Care Culture	**Traditional Care Culture**
Decentralized decision-making	Hierarchal decision-making
Empowered, multi-disciplinary teams	'Departmental' modality—staff follow instruction from supervisor
Adaptive and flexible organizational culture	Tightly managed organizational culture
Elders and staff design routines and schedules based on the elders preferences and needs	Routines and schedules based on organizational needs
Organizational culture does not fear making mistakes	Organizational culture does not acknowledge mistakes
Organizational culture values interpersonal, meaningful relationships with residents, staff, families and others	Organization culture values 'professional' distance from elders
Organizational culture addresses and resolves challenges as they occur	Organizational culture addresses challenges only when they become difficult to ignore
There is a sense of community and belonging	There is high structure and 'order'
Organization culture of continual assessment of outcomes	Organizational culture of sporadic assessment of outcomes
Low unintended staff turnover	Medium to high unintended staff turnover
Consistent staffing assignments	Rotating or varying staffing assignments
All levels of staff involved in problem-solving	Leadership/management involved in problem-solving
Organizational culture fosters continual staff learning culture and opportunities for professional training	Organizational culture mostly trains staff through in-services
All levels of staff involved in care/service planning	Management involved in care/service planning
All positions have the opportunity to spend time socializing with residents daily	Activity staff spend time socializing with residents
Organizational culture of spontaneous activities as well as arranged activities. Arranged activities are developed in conjunction with residents to ensure their preferences, interests, etc. are reflected.	Organizational culture of arranged activities conducted by activity staff

Source: Adapted from the Pioneer Network

Person-Centered Care Services

"For most dependent persons, quality care involves the emotional as well as physical realms and caters to personal needs and preferences, outcomes integrally tied to the nature of the caregiver-care receiver relationship (Ball et al., 2009). Person-centered care is focused on the emotional as well as the physical assistance to support normal daily life and optimize the well-being of the elders. Assistance with services such as activities of daily living (e.g., bathing, dressing, grooming) and dining are provided in a relationship-based context in which residents preferences,

146

interest and needs are learned through the interpersonal relationships. Staff, for example, become familiar with each resident's preferred daily routines and know when a resident prefers a warm evening shower and cup of tea before going to sleep. Person-centered care service is both the provision of external assistance, in this case the shower and cup of tea, and interpersonal relationships.

With person-centered care oriented services, staff encourage residents to do as much as possible for themselves so that they retain maximum independence and functioning. Building upon the fact that staff personally know the residents and thus her or his capabilities, staff know what and how much assistance is needed such as squeezing the toothpaste onto a toothbrush because arthritic fingers are painful in the morning, or twisting a lipstick tube so the resident can apply her own lipstick.

Reported Examples of Client/Resident Services Management to Support Person-Centered Care—

- Staff knowing when individual residents like to perform household tasks like folding their own laundry and ensuring they have the opportunity to do so.
- Ensuring that medications are only administered to residents in their preferred location rather than by default in the dining room.
- Staff knowing about and accommodating individual preferences to eat a late breakfast even when this is beyond normal dining room serving times.

Person-Centered Care Engagement

The goal of person-centered engagement is to optimize residents' psychosocial well-being through experiences that provide purpose and meaning in their daily lives and foster connections between community members. Person-centered engagement has upended the traditional system of an activity director solely providing recreational activities, often in groups, for socialization (Love, 2007). Activities, socialization, and engagement also are realigned in person-centered care since all staff are engaged in socializing and engaging with residents as part of the relationship-based culture.

Person-centered care engagement is structured very differently than traditional long-term care activities that are typically developed by an 'activity director' or 'recreational specialist' who creates a monthly calendar of varied activities. In a traditional model, residents use the activity calendar to select from among the choices what activities they are interested in. The activity specialist may need to cajole some residents to get out and participate at times in activities, but otherwise the residents are free to choose what, if any, activities they want to participate in. Staff, other than the activity specialist, are not very involved in resident activities/engagement except perhaps staff working in dementia special care environments who may conduct some activities to 'keep the residents occupied.'

By contrast, person-centered care engagement develops through a more natural, organic process that includes involvement from everyone who works, visits, or lives in the assisted living residence—in other words, the assisted living residence community. The activity specialist's role is to facilitate conversations so that ideas and suggestions for activities are openly discussed and mutually agreed upon. The activity specialist may be responsible for coordinating and/or scheduling some of the activities, but others in the community are just as likely to do so. This dynamic is significant because it changes the equation from residents, family members and staff being passive participants in engagement to one in which they are actively involved and invested. For instance, in one discussion a resident said that she missed playing Gin Rummy. Two other residents and a staff member spoke up saying they loved playing cards and would play with her.

What constitutes meaning and purpose differs for each individual. Some people are content with solitary activities such as reading books or listening to music all day, while others need the stimulation of people and like being involved in groups. Others derive satisfaction and purpose from helping others.

Examples of Client/Resident Services to Support Person-Centered Engagement

- Materials such as games, playing cards, puzzles, travel magazines, and wii video activities among many other materials are readily available in the assisted living residence to foster spontaneous engagement.
- Staff know which residents like to be helpful with daily tasks that could use their assistance such as setting out silverware and glasses, filling salt and pepper shakers, and folding towels and napkins to name a few.
- Young children are encouraged to visit and the assisted living residence has things available that are fun for children to use such as a toys or an outdoor play area.
- Dogs are encouraged to visit and the receptionist keeps a jar full of dog biscuits at the ready.

Person-Centered Care and NAB's Domain for Physical Environment Management

NAB Definition—Ensuring an environment and atmosphere that promotes, protects, and provides resident centered care and quality of life.

Person-Centered Care Environment & Design

A number of terms are used to describe the environment where assisted living residents live. Proponents of person-centered care recommend the term 'home' as most appropriate instead of terms such as 'home-like' or 'homey.' Since it is home for the residents, that term fits best. Beyond the physical bricks and mortar, person-centered care environments incorporate an emotional atmosphere created through design, use of space, colors, sound, furniture, furnishings and outdoor space.

The process of creating home requires evaluating the environment from a resident's perspective such as: what types of furniture groupings are comfortable and accessible; are the home's decorations meaningful to its residents; is lighting strong enough for aging eyes; is the atmosphere welcoming for visitors. Person-centered care environments and design are focused on comfort and personalization while also attentive to safety and accessibility issues.

Person-centered care physical environments are focused on features needed to support changes in elders' physical function and sensory losses including: short hallways and conveniently placed seating for those who tire quickly; shower areas in private bathrooms instead of bathtubs that are easier and safer to access; and flat doorway thresholds and shower areas without a lip to help prevent falls. Other common design considerations that are also consistent with person-centered care include increased lighting and amount of lighting; appropriate carpet designs so that patterns are not confusing; and the ability to smell foods they are cooking.

Some proponents of person-centered care are designing smaller, more intimate physical settings that are residential in scale. There are a number of these small home models including GREEN HOUSE®/assisted living, Households, and Cottages. Some of these models require new construction such as the GREEN HOUSE®/assisted living models, while others can be achieved through renovation, remodeling or retrofitting existing buildings. The small home models range in size from 4 to 16 residents. Besides providing for more home environments, the smaller settings are better able to foster individuals getting to know each other and forming home communities than larger settings.

Reported Examples of Physical Environment Management to Support Person-Centered Care—

- Residents are encouraged to add to the home's common area décor with some of their personal items ranging from a throw pillow and wall hanging to a curio or rocking chair.
- The use of natural sunlight is utilized as much as possible to keep interior spaces warm and welcoming.
- TV's in common areas are not left running throughout the day and instead are on only for specific programs.
- Gentle music plays in the dining room as meals are being served.

GLOSSARY

Choice: The act of selecting or choosing is a core value of assisted living.

Culture: A shared, learned, symbolic system of values, beliefs and attitudes that shapes and influences perception and behavior.

Dignity: A moral, ethical innate right to age appropriate respect and ethical treatment is a core value in assisted living.

Independence: As a core value of assisted living it is a freedom from control or influence of another or others. It is the ability to have direction of ones own affairs without interference.

Person-centered care: An empowering philosophy of care that rebalances work priorities from a focus on accomplishing tasks to a focus on the person needing assistance and optimizing their well-being.

Privacy: The right of the resident to seclude himself or his information and the right to reveal information if and when that person chooses to have it revealed. This is one of the core values of RC/AL.

Respect: A core value of assisted living that is to treat each resident with courtesy, consideration, and kindness.

PRACTICE QUESTIONS

Read each item carefully, and then select the best response.

1. For most staff their primary component of job satisfaction is:
   A. their relationships with residents.
   B. mentoring of fellow co-workers.
   C. ability to have personal growth.
   D. praise and recognition from administrator.

   A B C D
   ○ ○ ○ ○

2. Person-centered care in the field of aging:
   A. is built around staffing convenience.
   B. focuses on accomplishing tasks.
   C. revolves around an organizations structure.
   D. is a relationship-based philosophy.

   A B C D
   ○ ○ ○ ○

3. Studies show the estimated staff turnover for each direct care worker is:
   A. $1250.
   B. $1500.
   C. $2000.
   D. $2500.

   A B C D
   ○ ○ ○ ○

4. Person-centered care physical environments would include:
   A. soft, natural and relaxing lighting.
   B. carpet designs that are not confusing to residents.
   C. long hallways for wandering residents.
   D. bathtubs in each residents private bathroom.

   A B C D
   ○ ○ ○ ○

5. Rather than a regimented diagram of staff responsibilities person-centered care leadership:
   A. allows staff to make mistakes from which they can learn.
   B. will definitely improve morale and efficiency of staff.
   C. can add organization to the staff responsibilities while improving performance.
   D. empowers staff to improve resident satisfaction by assigning specific duties to specific staff.

   A B C D
   ○ ○ ○ ○

6. Which of the below is *not* an example of person centered care?
   A. Rotating or varying staffing assignments to learn about each resident
   B. The facility has a tradition of how to welcome new residents
   C. The RC/AL community has a custom of how to acknowledge the death of a resident
   D. Staff regularly eat meals with residents to give the opportunity to converse and connect

   A B C D
   ○ ○ ○ ○

7. Principles of individuality and choice require services to be tailored to each individuals unique preferences and circumstances. This personalization is reflected in:
   A. the physicians assessment.
   B. the residents medical record.
   C. the residents plan of services.
   D. the negotiated risk agreement.

A B C D
○ ○ ○ ○

8. While there is no common barometer for measuring what constitutes quality of person-centered care, most agree:
   A. all residents deserve individualized attention.
   B. staff should treat residents as family members.
   C. all staff should increase and promote individual interaction.
   D. well-being is the desired outcome.

A B C D
○ ○ ○ ○

9. Person-centered care culture has:
   A. a tightly managed organizational structure.
   B. decentralized decision making.
   C. medium to high unintended staff turnover.
   D. rotating or varying staff assignments.

A B C D
○ ○ ○ ○

10. Traditional care culture has:
    A. adaptive and flexible organizational structure.
    B. a sense of community and belonging.
    C. routines based on organizational needs.
    D. all levels of staff involved in problem-solving.

A B C D
○ ○ ○ ○

ANSWERS AND EXPLANATIONS

1. **Correct answer = A.** "It is through their relationships with residents that staff find meaning in these . . . jobs. For most (staff), their relationships with residents are the primary component of job satisfaction (Ball et al., 2009)."

2. **Correct answer = D.** The power and value of relationships cannot be overstated. Person centered care is an empowering philosophy of care that rebalances work priorities from a focus on accomplishing tasks to a focus on the person needing assistance.

3. **Correct answer = D.** $2500! This amount only includes the direct costs associated with recruiting and training new staff. One report estimated that in a typical RC/AL the annual impact is $84,537.

4. **Correct answer = B.** Person centered care physical environments are focused on features needed to support changes in residents physical function and sensory loss.

5. **Correct answer = A.** Person centered care ushers in a transformed organizational chart structure that is circular. Allowing staff to make mistakes from which they can learn will foster empowerment and engagement.

6. **Correct answer = A.** Consistent staffing allows for staff to become familiar with the residents typical behaviors, moods, and appearances while also developing the relationships with them.

7. **Correct answer = C.** This personalization is reflected in a plan of services negotiated with the resident (and/or her representative) that specifies how and what services are to be provided.

8. **Correct answer = D.** Person centered care focuses both on quality of life and quality of care with the goal of optimizing resident well-being.

9. **Correct answer = B.** Person centered care culture has decentralized decision making as opposed to traditional culture. Decentralization decision-making occurs when leaders empower staff to address and make decisions related to their work responsibilities.

10. **Correct answer = C.** Traditional culture has routines and schedules based on organizational needs as opposed to person centered care culture in which schedules are based on residents preferences and needs.

REFERENCES

Ball, M.M., Lepore, M.L., Perkins, M.M., Hollingsworth, C., Sweatman, M. (2009). "They are the reason I come to work": The meaning of resident-staff relationships in assisted living. Journal of Aging Studies. 23:37-47.

Barry, T., Brannon, D., Mor, V. 2005. Nurse aide empowerment strategies and staff stability: Effects on nursing home resident outcomes. *The Gerontolo*gist. 45(3), 309-317.

Bowers, B. 2009. Implementing change in long-term care: A practical guide to transformation. Prepared by The Commonwealth Fund. New York, New York: The Commonwealth Fund.

Castle, N.G., Engbert, J. 2006. Organizational characteristics associated with staff turnover in nursing homes. *The Gerontologist*. 46(1), 62-73.

Donoghue, C., Castle, N.G. 2009. Leadership styles of nursing home administrators and their association with staff turnover. *The Gerontologist*. 49(2), 166-174.

Fazio, S. 2008. Person-centered care in residential settings: Taking a look back while continuing to move forward. *Alzheimer's Care Today*. 9(2), 155-161.

Ferrell, D., Dawson, S. 2007. The business case for investing in staff retention: can you afford not to? *futureAge*. 3, 8-11.

Frampton, S.B., Gilpin, L., Charmel, P.A. 2003. Putting Patients First: Designing and

Practicing Patient-Centered Care. San Francisco: John Wiley & Sons, Inc.

Holleran, M.D. 2007. Six key leadership behaviors that support culture change. A White Paper prepared by the American Association of Homes and Services for the Aging. Washington, DC: American Association of Homes and Services for the Aging. Online at www.aahsa.org.

Hyde, J., Perez, R., Reed, P.S. 2008. The old road is rapidly aging: A social model for cognitively or physically impaired elders in assisted living's future. In Golant, S. M. & Hyde, J. (Eds.), *The assisted living residence: A vision for the future* (pp. 46-85). Baltimore: Johns Hopkins University Press.

Jacob, B. 2002. Using a mission statement to staff assisted living. *Nursing Homes Magazine.* 51, 54-57.

Kane, R.A., Wilson, K.B. 1998. Assisted living in the united states: A new paradigm for residential care. Prepared by AARP. Washington, DC: AARP.

Kantor, B., Elliot, A., Frank, B., Brady, C., Farrell, D., McLaughlin, M. (2009) Culture change and resident centered care: Addendum to the NAB nursing home administrators examination study guide. A paper prepared by the Pioneer Network. Rochester, New York: Pioneer Network.

Keane, B. 2005. The death of culture change. *Nursing Homes Management.* 54(11), 30-33.

Kemp, C.L., Ball, M.M., Perkins, M.M., Hollingsworth, C., Lepore, M.J. 2009. "I get along with most of them": Direct care workers' relationships with residents' families in assisted living. *The Gerontologist.* 49(2), 224-235.

Kiefer, K.M., Harris-Kojetin, L., Brannon, D., Barry, T., Vasey, J., Lepore, M. April, 2005. *Measuring long-term care work: A guide to selected instruments to examine direct care worker experiences and outcomes.* Prepared by the U.S. Department of Health and Human Services and the U.S. Department of Labor. Washington, DC: U.S. Department of Health and Human Services.

Love, K. 2007. Montessori techniques: Not just child's play. *Assisted Living Consult.* 3(6), 21-24.

Lustbader, W., Williams, C.C. 2006. Culture change in long-term care. In Berkman, A. & D'Ambruoso, S. (Eds.), *Handbook of Social Work in Health and Aging* (pp. 645-652). New York: Oxford University Press.

PHI, & Institute for the Future of Aging Services. January, 2005. *Workforce Strategies—No. 3.* Prepared by PHI & Institute for the Future of Aging Services. New York, New York: PHI.

Pratt, J.R. 2004. *Long-term care, second edition: Managing across the continuum.* Sudbury: Jones and Bartlett Publishers, Inc.

Seavey, D. 2004. *The cost of frontline turnover in long-term care.* Better Jobs Better Care. Washington, DC: The Institute for the Future of Aging Services.

Sikorska-Simmons, E. 2005. Predictors of organizational commitment among staff in assisted living. *The Gerontologist.* 45(2), 196-205.

Smull, M.W. 2000. Listen, learn, act: Selected writings by Michael W. Smull on essential lifestyle planning, self-determination, and organizational change. Online at www.elpnet.net/home.html.

Wiener, J.M., Stevenson, D.G., Goldenson, S.M. 1999. Controlling the supply of long-term care providers in thirteen states. *Journal of Aging, Society and Policy.* 10(4), 51-72.

Wilson, K. B. 1995. Assisted living as a model of care delivery. In Gamroth, L.M., Semradeck, J., & Tornquist, E.M. (Eds.), *Enhancing Autonomy in Long-term Care* (pp. 139—54). New York: Springer.

Wilson, K. B. 2007. Historical evolution of assisted living in the united states, 1979 to the present. The Gerontologist 47 (Supplement):8-22

Zimmerman, S., Sloane, P.D., Fletcher, S.K. 2008. The measurement and importance of quality. In Golant, S. M. & Hyde, J.

(Eds.), *The assisted living residence: A vision for the future* (pp. 119-142). Baltimore: Johns Hopkins University Press.

Resources for Person-Centered Care

Websites

- Better Jobs Better Care—www.bjbc.org
- The GREEN HOUSE Replication Project— www.thegreenhouseproject.org
- IDEAS (Innovative Designs in Environment for an Aging Society) Consulting—www.ideasconsultinginc.com.
- The National Clearinghouse on the Direct Care Workforce—www.directcareclearinghouse.org
- The Pioneer Network—www.pioneernetwork.net
- Planetree—www.planetree.org

Literature

- Ball, M.M., Lepore, M.L., Perkins, M.M., Hollingsworth, C., Sweatman, M. (2009). "They are the reason I come to work": The meaning of resident-staff relationships in assisted living. Journal of Aging Studies. 23:37-47.
- Brawley, Elizabeth (1997). Designing for Alzheimer's Desease: Strategies for Creating Better Care Environments. New York: Wiley & Sons.
- Buckingham, M., & Coffman, C. (1999). First, Break All the Rules: What the World's Greatest Managers Do Differently. New York: Simon & Schuster.
- Edmondson, A.C. (2008). The competitive imperative of learning. *Harvard Business Review*. July-August hbr.org.
- Gladwell, M. (2002). The Tipping Point: How Little Things Can Make a Big Difference. Boston: Little Brown.
- Garvin, D.A., Edmondson, A.C., Gino, F. (2008). Is yours a learning organization? *Harvard Business Review*. March hbr.org.
- Kotter, J. (1996). Leading Change. Cambridge: Harvard University Press.
- Murphey, E., & Joffe, S. (2001). Creating a Culture of Retention: A Coaching Approach to Paraprofessional Supervision. New York: Paraprofessional Healthcare Institute.
- Noelker, L.S., & Harel, Z., (Eds.) (2000). Linking Quality of Long-Term Care and Quality of Life. New York: Springer Publishing Company, Inc.
- Sloane, P.D., Brooker, D., Cohen, L., Douglass, C., Edelman, P., Fulton, R.G., Jarrott, S., Kasayka, R., Kuhn, D., Preisser, J.S., Williams, C.S., Zimmerman, S. (2007). Dementia care mapping as a research tool. *International Journal of Geriatric Psychiatry*, 22(6):580-589.

Disclaimer of Endorsement: Reference herein to any trademark, proprietary product, or company name is intended for explicit description only and does not constitute or imply endorsement or recommendation by the NAB, or anyone else.